BEAUTY FROM THE INSIDE OUT

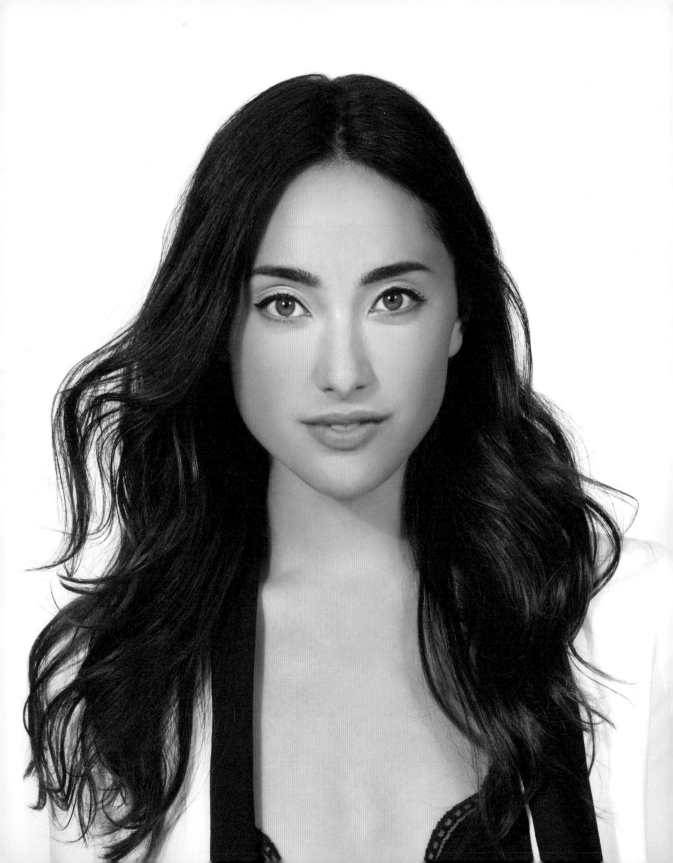

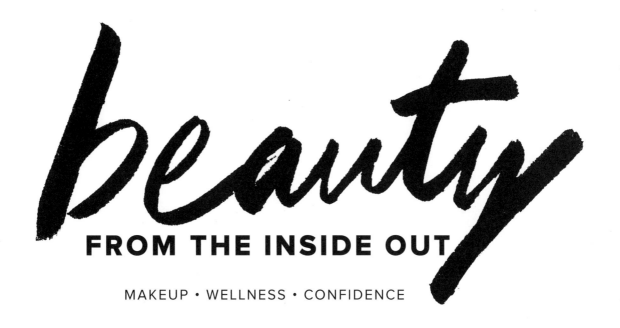

beauty

FROM THE INSIDE OUT

MAKEUP · WELLNESS · CONFIDENCE

BOBBI BROWN

with SARA BLISS

CHRONICLE BOOKS

SAN FRANCISCO

Library of Congress Cataloging-in-Publication Data

Names: Brown, Bobbi, author.
Title: Bobbi Brown's beauty from the inside out / Bobbi Brown.
Description: San Francisco : Chronicle Books, [2017] | Includes index.
Identifiers: LCCN 2016042342 | ISBN 9781452161846 (hardback)
Subjects: LCSH: Nutrition—Popular works. | Diet—Popular works. | Beauty, Personal—Popular works. | BISAC: HEALTH & FITNESS / Beauty & Grooming. | HEALTH & FITNESS / Healthy Living.
Classification: LCC RA784 .B74 2017 | DDC 613.2—dc23 LC record available at https://lccn.loc.gov/2016042342

Manufactured in China.

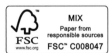

Design by Pamela Geismar.

10 9 8 7 6 5 4 3 2

Chronicle Books LLC
680 Second Street
San Francisco, California 94107
www.chroniclebooks.com

Chronicle books and gifts are available at special quantity discounts to corporations, professional associations, literacy programs, and other organizations. For details and discount information, please contact our corporate/premiums department at corporatesales@chroniclebooks.com or at 1-800-759-0190.

contents

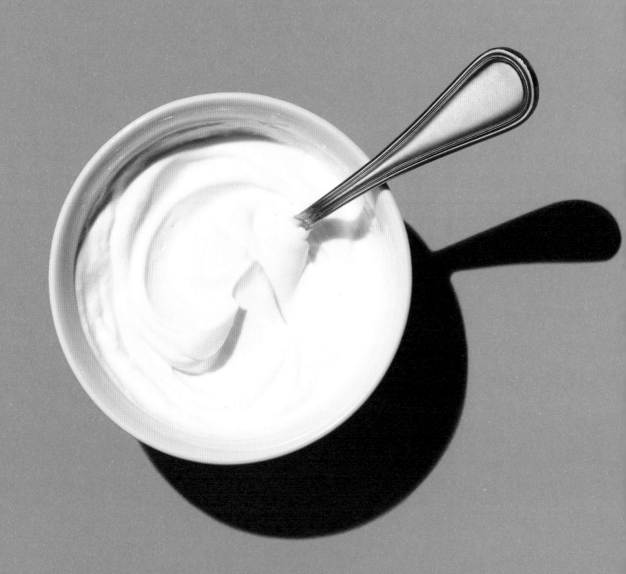

INTRODUCTION

When it comes to beauty, I'm a firm believer that it starts from the inside out. For me, it's simple: Your health shows on your face. If you take care of yourself—by eating the healthiest foods possible, drinking a ton of water, and moving your body every day—it shows. You look good and you feel good. You're comfortable and confident in your own skin.

But I also know that life happens. There are times of stress, travel, late nights, and fluctuating hormones when you may not look or feel your best. I understand because it happens to me all the time. This is why the right skincare and makeup can be confidence-savers. My approach to beauty on the outside has always been centered on healthy skin and a natural glow.

Everyone's journey to health, wellness, and beauty is different. That's why I wrote this book with a little help from my friends—to offer the inspiration, products, and tips that will help you be the best version of yourself from the inside out.

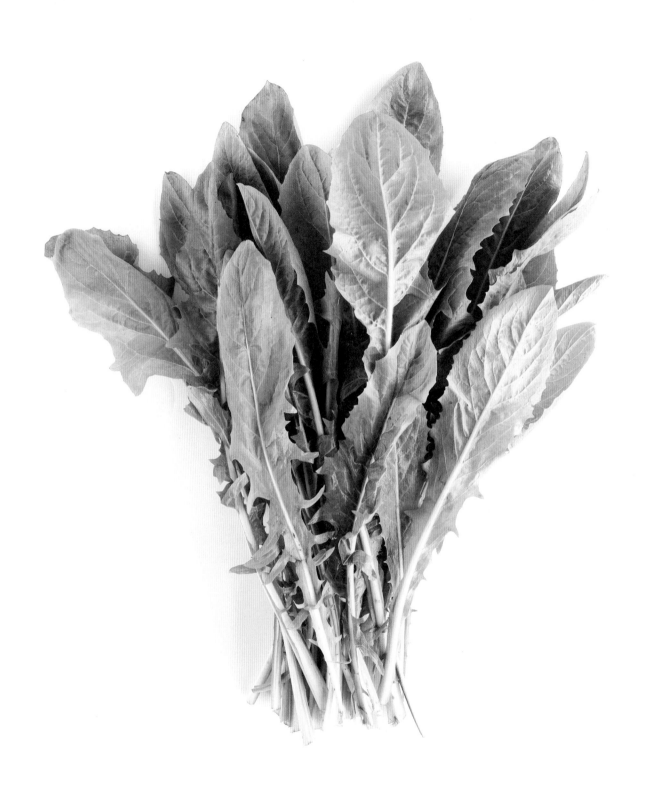

1 Beauty Food

The link between beauty and food wasn't something I always understood. I was a health nut in the '80s and '90s. I collected a library of fad diet books and was convinced that each one had the answer to good health and the perfect body. There was the Beverly Hills Diet (fruit only before noon), Pritikin (no fat and lots of whole grains), Scarsdale (lots of steak and eggs), and then Atkins (tons of high-fat foods like meat, bacon, and cheese, but not a lot of fruits or vegetables). My goal was to lose weight and lose it quickly. But losing pounds by eating unhealthy foods didn't work and didn't make me feel good.

I began to make the connection that the foods I was eating were making me feel slow and tired. After a bagel my energy would crash. I stopped eating cookies, bread, and pasta and immediately felt better. I started paying attention. I noticed I felt great when I drank a lot of water, so I started to count my glasses and tried to drink at least eight per day. I felt better when I ate fruits that were not too sweet. The fresher and more simply prepared the produce, the better my digestion. I started eating my veggies steamed and drizzled with good olive oil. Soon I had more energy and better focus, my skin looked healthier, and my eyes were clearer. I was on to something.

I ditched the weight loss books and began to read about health and wellness, discovering doctors, chiropractors, and nutritionists who practiced whole-body health. Since then, I've shifted my lifestyle, paying closer attention to what goes into my body. For eating out, I'm excited by cool restaurants that serve real local foods. At home, I can whip up a simple, fast meal using nutritious ingredients that's robust enough to feed a family of boys. Health food is life food—and ultimately beauty food.

The cornerstone of beauty foods are fresh vegetables and fruits that provide your fuel, good fats like omega-3s for skin and health, and lean proteins that provide energy. By eating a diet balanced in these types of nutrient-rich foods most of the time, you will feel and look better.

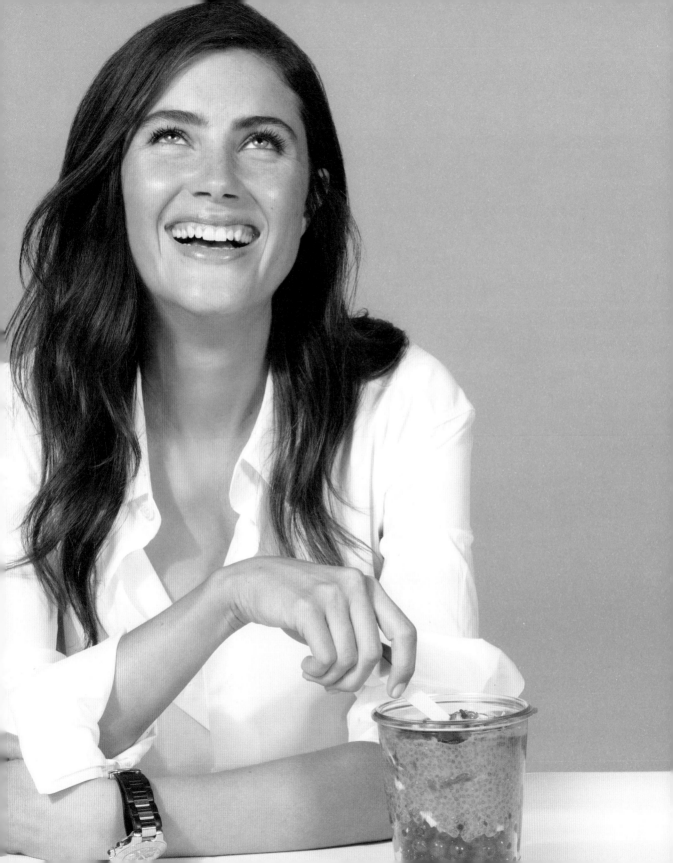

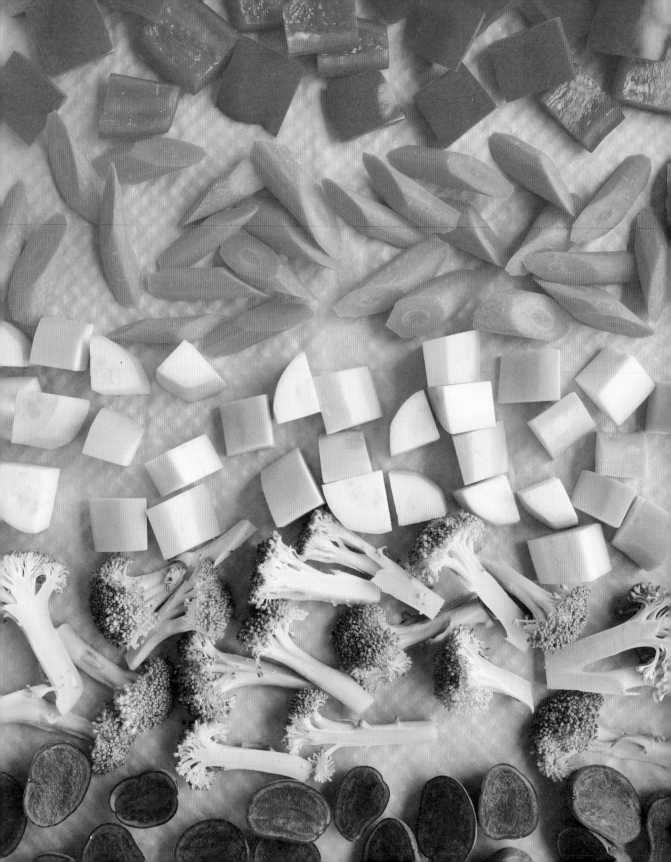

beauty superfoods

———

Not only can the right foods increase your energy, prevent disease, and keep you healthy, they can also make you look great. When you eat foods that are packed with nutrients, you will see a difference.

Nutritionist Dr. Charles Passler has taught me a lot about food and health. I asked him to share his ultimate list of beauty superfoods. The list contains the building blocks and nutrients needed for healthy tissue support, development, and protection. "Fats and proteins are required to provide healthy tissue development, especially collagen. Nutrients called antioxidants (such as vitamins A, C, E, and zinc and selenium) provide protection against free radicals and the damage created from too much sun," explains Dr. Passler. "It is also important to choose foods that support digestive health. Without proper breakdown, absorption, and removal of waste by the digestive system, it is impossible for your body to provide the support needed for healthy eyes, hair, nails, and skin."

Passler notes that hydration, sleep, and exercise are essential pieces of the puzzle. "It is impossible for your cells to be healthy and vibrant without proper hydration," he explains. "Sweating is a great way to keep your pores clean and to be sure that your circulation is optimized so that every cell gets the necessary support. Sleeping is when the majority of cellular healing and repair and detoxification occur. Adequate sleep is a must."

Dr. Passler's Beauty Superfoods:

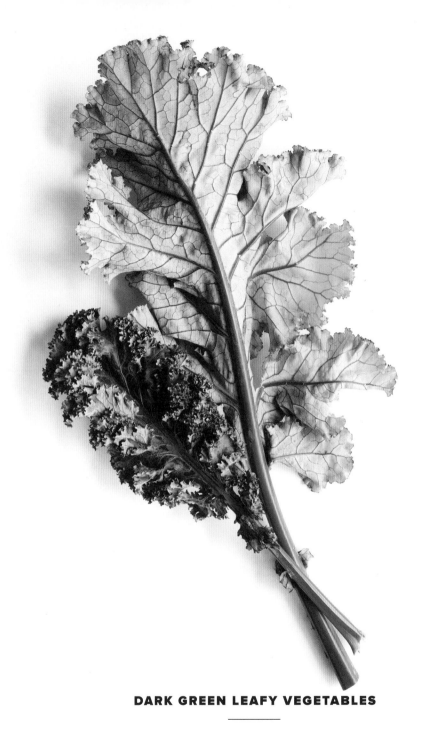

DARK GREEN LEAFY VEGETABLES

Kale, alfalfa, and spinach are wonderful for skin. They support and increase collagen production. They are also full of antioxidants.

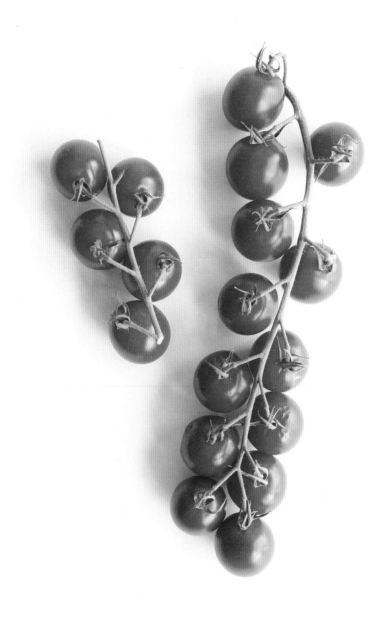

RED VEGETABLES

Tomatoes, red peppers, and beets help improve collagen formation and contain lycopene to protect the cells from free radical damage and from the damaging rays of the sun, making them a natural sunblock.

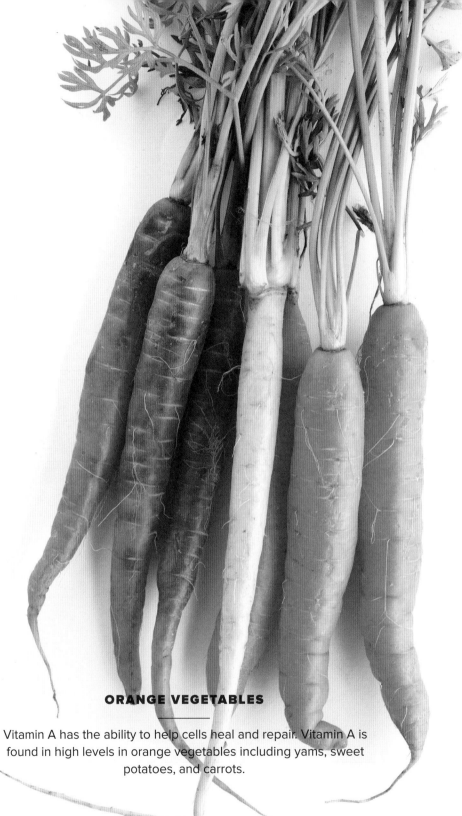

ORANGE VEGETABLES

Vitamin A has the ability to help cells heal and repair. Vitamin A is found in high levels in orange vegetables including yams, sweet potatoes, and carrots.

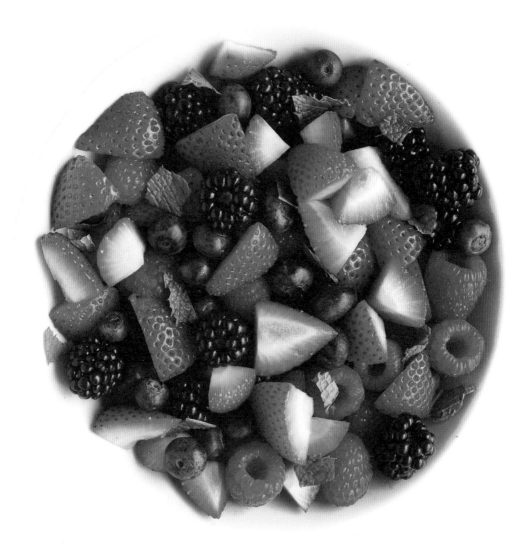

BLUEBERRIES AND RASPBERRIES

Loaded with antioxidants, these dark berries improve collagen
production.

CITRUS AND TROPICAL FRUITS

Lemons, limes, grapefruit, oranges, mangos, guavas, and papayas all have high levels of the powerful antioxidant vitamin C and will protect cells against free radicals. They also play a role in the formation of collagen.

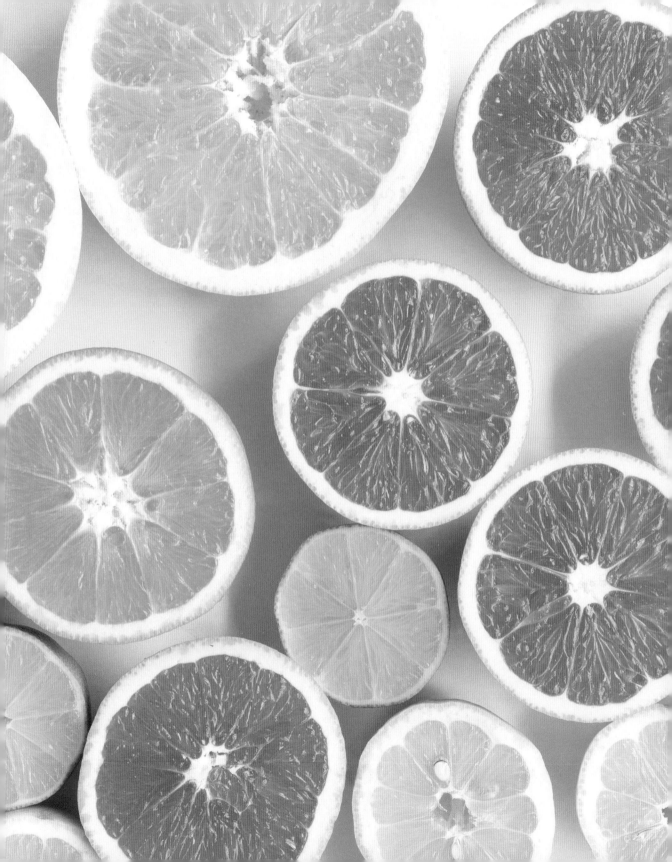

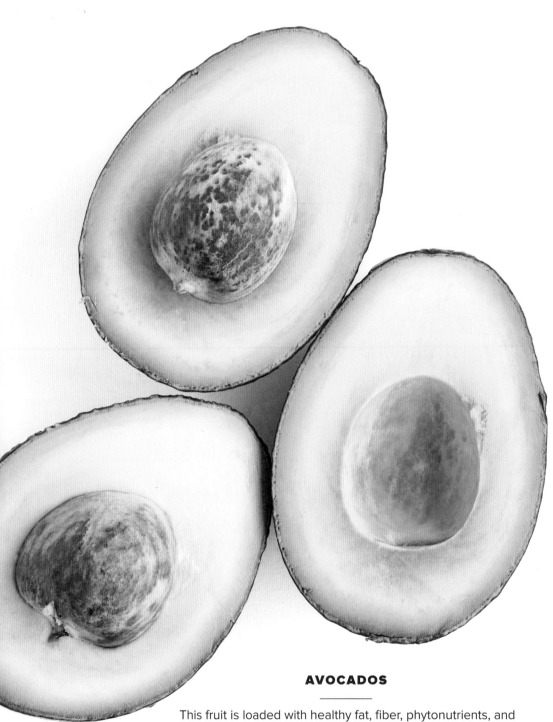

AVOCADOS

This fruit is loaded with healthy fat, fiber, phytonutrients, and antioxidants. The antioxidants have a protective benefit and the fiber is great for digestive health.

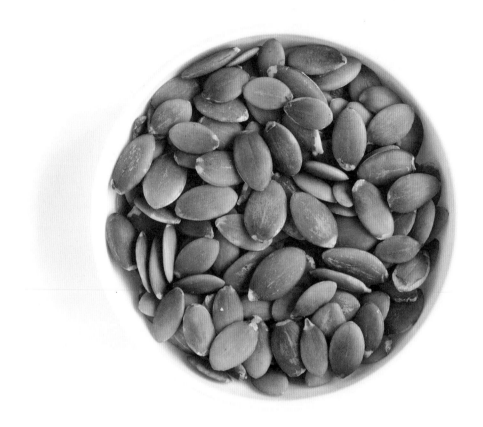

PUMPKIN SEEDS

These seeds are high in zinc, which protects cell membranes and helps maintain and produce collagen. Zinc also helps fight breakouts.

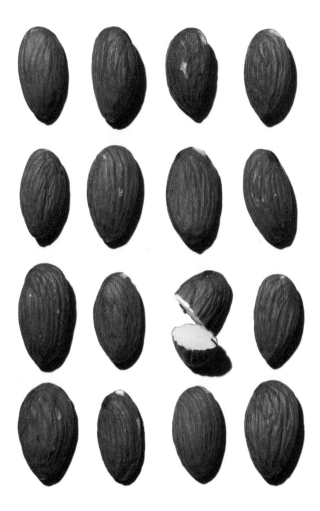

RAW ALMONDS

These nuts are high in the antioxidant vitamin E, which is crucial for smooth, healthy skin. They are also wonderful sources of protein.

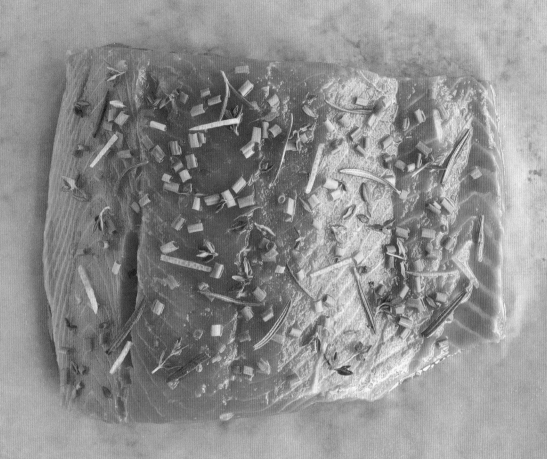

FISH OIL

Wild Alaskan salmon and sardines are both very high in omega-3 oil, which creates stronger cells by supporting the protective fatty membranes around skin cells. For the non-fish-eater, flax and chia seeds are good alternative sources of omega-3s.

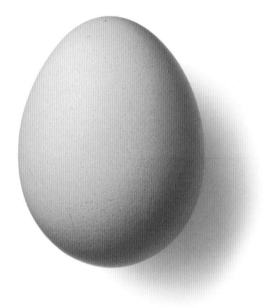

EGGS

Eggs are loaded with protein and fats that help support the production of collagen. Eggs are also a good source of vitamin A, which helps cells repair and reboot. Cooked eggs, particularly the yolks, offer almost a full RDA (recommended dietary allowance) of biotin, a nutrient essential for healthy hair and nails.

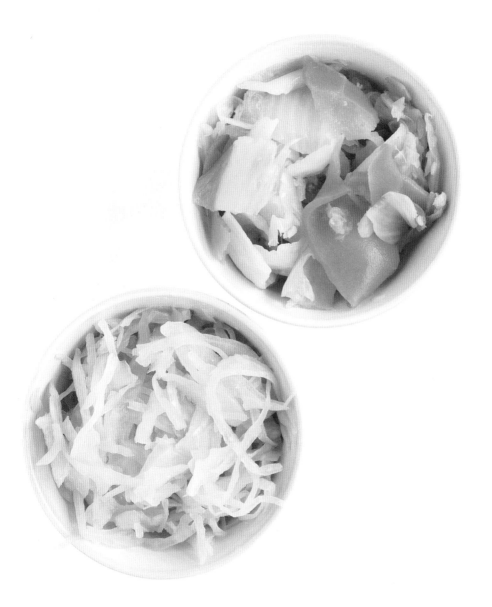

FERMENTED FOODS

Sauerkraut, kimchi, kombucha, yogurt, and kefir are all fermented foods loaded with live bacteria, known as probiotics, that will boost your digestive system, allowing for improved absorption of nutrients, increased detoxification, decreased inflammation, improved immune function, and balanced hormones, all of which help with eye, hair, nail, and skin health. A healthy digestive system can also help with losing weight. Be sure that the products you choose are not pasteurized, as pasteurization destroys the health benefits of live bacteria.

BOLD COLORS = HEALTHY FOOD

I am color obsessed so I am automatically drawn to fruits and vegetables in vibrant hues. The cool thing is that often the more intense the color, the healthier the food. Beauty foods that are packed with nutrients come in bold reds, rich purples and pinks, deep greens, vivid yellows and oranges, and strong blues. Let color guide you the next time you are shopping at a farmers' market or grocery store. And when you are putting together a plate of food, think as much about eating a variety of colors as types of food. Each color group features different nutrients, so the more variation you have, the more balanced the meal. Create plates filled with a variety of colors, textures, and tastes.

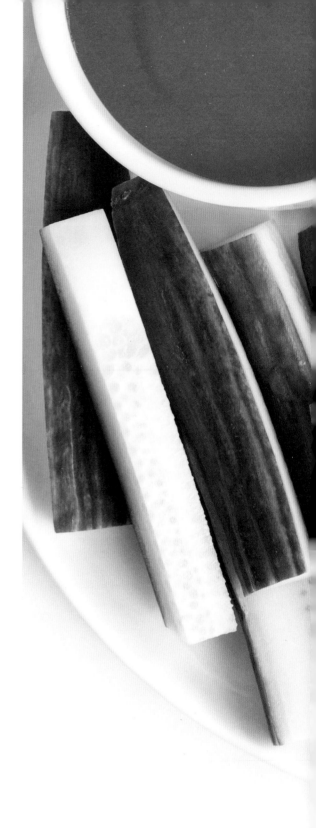

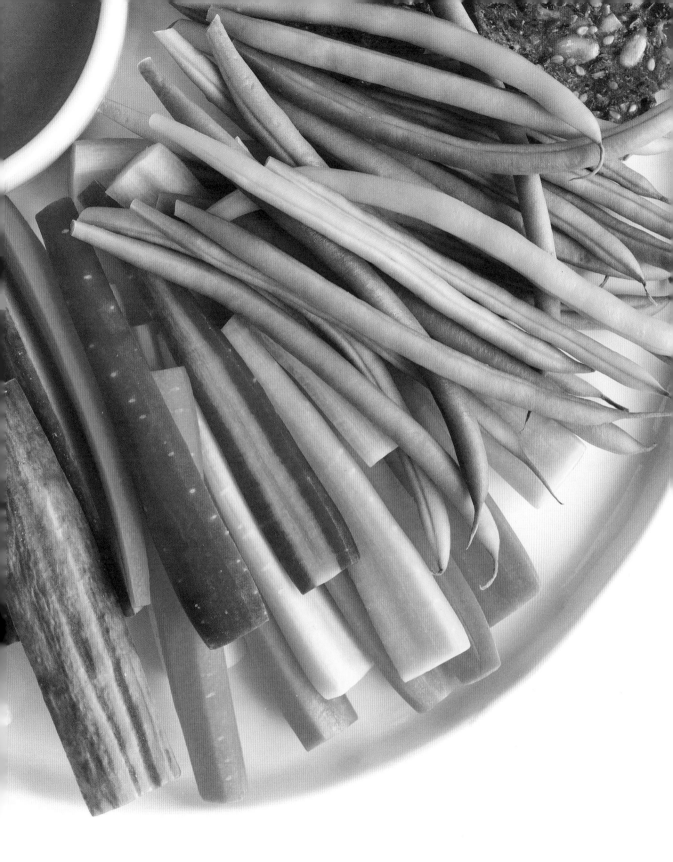

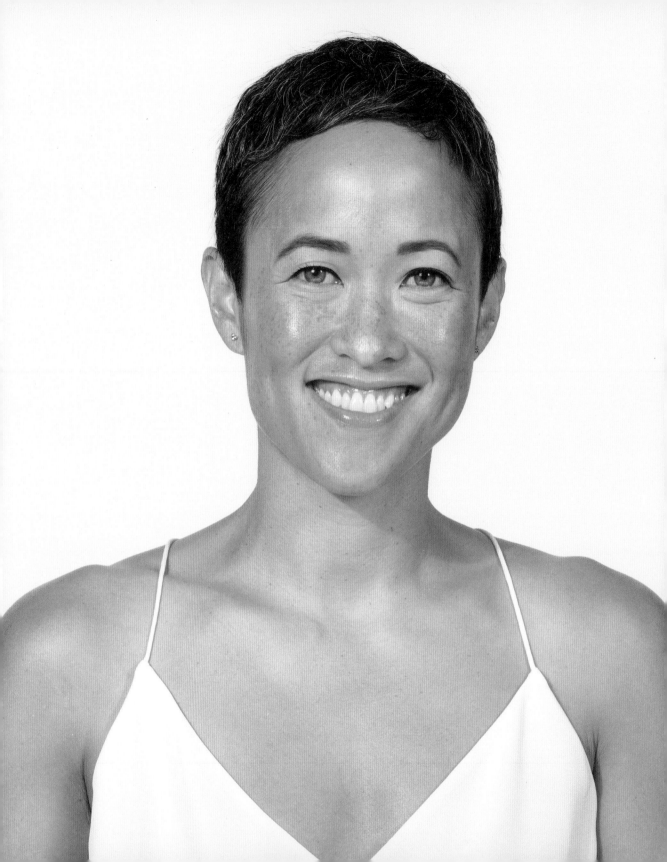

my beauty food essentials

Over the years, I've found my best foods for increased energy and beautiful skin. I make a point to try to eat what is fresh and in season. I love to stock up at the farmers' market or pick from my backyard garden, where I plant tomatoes, kale, cucumbers, zucchini, and lots of fresh herbs.

APPLE CIDER VINEGAR: This is an ingredient nearly everyone has in their kitchen, but it also doubles as a health and beauty remedy helping to reduce bloating, clear skin, and make the body more alkaline. To consume, mix one small spoonful with a glass of water.

BERRIES: Blueberries, blackberries, and raspberries are full of fiber and antioxidants. They are sweet enough to satisfy a sugar craving and you can sprinkle them with cinnamon to create a favorite dessert of mine.

FLAXSEED, HEMP SEEDS, CHIA SEEDS: I put these seeds into pretty much everything—smoothies, oatmeal, and desserts. They are all full of protein, fiber, and omega-3s.

HYDRATING FOODS: Another way to hydrate is to eat foods with a high water content. Cucumber is 96 percent water (the highest water content of any solid food). Other foods that are more than 90 percent water include tomatoes, watermelon, and radishes.

GREEN POWDERS: A scoop of green nutrient powder mixed with a glass of water is a great way to start the day and make my system more alkaline and less acidic. My favorite powders right now are WelleCo's Super Elixir Alkalising Greens and AlkaMind Daily Greens. They give me that extra burst of energy and are packed with foods and nutrients I may not get every day, such as wheatgrass, dandelion leaf, chlorophyll, chlorella, and sprouts.

ORGANIC WHEY POWDER: This super-clean protein is a go-to for me. I put it in a shaker bottle with water or coconut or almond milk. I also make a mean protein-filled hot cocoa with chocolate whey, coconut milk, cacao, cinnamon, and a sprinkle of ground red pepper for kick. Tera's Whey is my favorite.

VEGETABLES: The majority of my diet is vegetables. I eat a ton of salads, raw veggies as snacks, and steamed vegetables as sides. I add frozen spinach and kale (both filled with antioxidants and fiber) to my morning smoothies. I also drink green juice when I need an afternoon pick-me-up— it works better than caffeine.

WATER: Water is a game changer for your body, brain, and beauty. Your skin looks more plump and fresh when you are hydrated. Water also flushes out toxins, which seriously improves the appearance of your skin.

LEMONS: Lemon juice mixed into a glass of water cleanses, alkalizes, and adds an immunity-boosting dose of vitamin C. Before you eat break-fast, squeeze half a lemon into a glass of water to get the maximum benefits.

PEPPERMINT: Great for digestion and vitality, peppermint is a refreshing touch when infused in water, sprinkled on fruit, or blended into smoothies.

COCONUT OIL: Rich in good saturated fats that are great for health and skin, coconut oil also reduces inflammation. To work it into your diet, mix it into a smoothie, cook with it, or drink a spoonful daily.

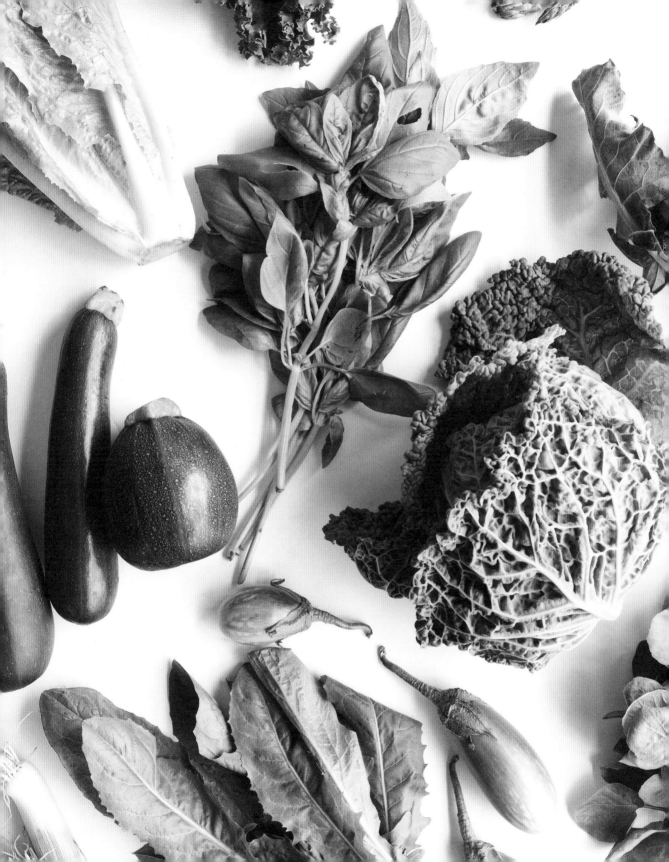

eat beautiful: nutrient chart

———

Knowing what foods contain which nutrients will help you balance out your diet. This way you can also target specific beauty concerns by eating foods rich in the nutrients you need. To understand which major vitamins and minerals amp up beauty, I turned to health coach Linda Arrandt and nutritionist and alkaline diet expert Daryl Gioffre.

NUTRIENT	WHAT IT DOES	WHAT TO EAT
CAROTENOIDS	These highly pigmented foods rich in vitamin A can affect skin color, creating a natural, healthy glow from within.	Red peppers, pumpkin, carrots, apricots, cantaloupe, sweet potatoes, broccoli, and leafy greens.
LYCOPENE	Boosts skin's natural SPF.	Tomatoes, watermelon, pink grapefruit, and red peppers.
POTASSIUM	An essential mineral for neutralizing toxins and acidity. Also fights puffiness.	Bananas, beet greens, Swiss chard, sweet potatoes, avocados, and cooked lentils.
VITAMIN A	Helps cells repair and renew, making it a must for keeping skin young and vibrant. Also excellent for eye health, which is key since everyone's eyesight starts to diminish after age 40.	Sweet potatoes and yams are the best source, followed by carrots, butternut squash, kale, and spinach.
VITAMIN B2 (RIBOFLAVIN)	Boosts metabolism and reduces inflammation. Maintains eye health.	Lamb will provide 100 percent of your daily requirement. Almonds, avocados, beets, and mushrooms are other good sources.

NUTRIENT	WHAT IT DOES	WHAT TO EAT
VITAMIN B7 (BIOTIN)	Supports healthy and strong hair and nails.	Almonds, sweet potatoes, egg yolks, and avocado. If you are experiencing hair loss, a biotin supplement may help.
VITAMIN B8 (FOLATE)	Excellent for hair growth and cell healing.	Garbanzo beans are the best source, followed by lentils, pinto beans, and asparagus.
VITAMIN C	Excellent for keeping skin glowing, as it increases collagen production.	Oranges, grapefruit, kiwis, spinach, red and green peppers, Brussels sprouts, and cantaloupe.
VITAMIN E	An anti-aging powerhouse, vitamin E helps maintain youthful, hydrated, elastic skin and provides a moisture boost to hair as well. The antioxidant helps to heal acne and scarring.	Sunflower seeds, almonds, hazelnuts, spinach, asparagus, and avocado.
VITAMIN K	Boosts bone density, helps with blood clotting, and strengthens blood vessels.	Spinach, dandelion greens, kale, broccoli, and Brussels sprouts.
ZINC	Helps prevent breakouts and promotes clear skin. Also boosts immunity.	Lentils, pumpkin seeds, and kidney beans.

beauty-zapping foods

While some foods make you look and feel better, there are many others that can do the opposite. "When we eat anything with sugar or flour, especially if we do it on a daily basis or multiple times a day, we spike our insulin, which causes us to store fat, spike our testosterone, or turn testosterone into estrogen, which can lead to weight gain and imbalances in hormones like PMS, fibroids, and endometriosis," explains Dr. Robin Berzin of Parsley Health. "You also age faster because oxidation leads to DNA damage, meaning damage of cell walls and cellular proteins." Thankfully, eating whole foods can actually reverse the clock. "If you are eating a diet rich in fiber and plants and all of those phytonutrients, those are going to fuel your body to make its own antioxidants," says Dr. Berzin. "You're going to repair damage and start looking and feeling younger, because your body will heal." Here's what to avoid:

PROCESSED FOODS: Most processed foods have a ton of preservatives, dyes, emulsifiers, and chemicals. "All of these are toxic to the body and can disrupt our hormone system and fatty acid metabolism. Fatty acids are important to balancing skin and giving it luster," explains Berzin. "When you eat processed foods, your body becomes overloaded trying to detoxify the chemicals in those foods. You don't look as good, feel as good, sleep as well, or have good digestion." Processed foods don't have the same amount of vitamins and minerals you get from eating whole foods. When you fill up on fake foods, you're losing the opportunity to get energy from food that truly fuels you from the inside.

SALT: The effects of too much salt can be seen almost immediately. Eat a meal that's heavy in sodium and you'll wake up looking puffy and swollen, especially around the eyes. And it doesn't just affect your face: excess salt can increase water retention in the body. Fast food, processed food, and salty snacks are obvious culprits, but watch out for canned soups, salad dressings, and bread, which can also contain large amounts of salt.

SODA: When you drink sugar, you are filling up on empty calories with zero nutritional value. Soda is filled with chemicals and incredibly high amounts of sugar or chemical sugar substitutes, both of which cause insulin spikes. To stay hydrated and eliminate toxins, you need to rely on water as your primary source of hydration. When you give up soda, you may also notice clearer skin.

SUGAR: Whether it's white sugar or high fructose corn syrup, sugar wreaks havoc on your body. It's incredibly addictive and causes your blood sugar to rise, which causes a host of problems, from energy crashes to hormonal imbalances. Sugar has been linked to a range of diseases, including cancer, diabetes, and obesity. It messes with gut health and can create an overgrowth of yeast and bad bacteria. It also damages collagen and elastin, causing skin to age more rapidly. Try coconut sugar as an alternative, as it has a lower glycemic index. However, the biggest boost is to radically reduce the amount of sugar you consume.

WHITE FLOUR: White flour, found in most bread and baked goods, has no nutritional value and causes blood sugar to spike. If you're trying to eat healthier or more alkaline, note that white flour is very acidic in the body. Try using oat or almond flour as alternatives.

ABOUT ALCOHOL

I love to have a cocktail or two and still stay healthy. So I asked nutritionist and founder of New York–based Foodtrainers, Lauren Slayton, how to understand the balance.

BEST ALCOHOLS TO DRINK: Spirits (tequila, vodka, Scotch) on the rocks or with club soda beat wine because of the lower sugar content.

HOW OFTEN: One drink a day for women, two for men. If there's any type of weight loss goal, modify to four or fewer drinks per week for women and seven or below for guys.

HOW TO BALANCE: Our rule is one for one. Drink a glass of water before you enjoy each cocktail.

AVOID A HANGOVER: Alcohol depletes you. Vitamins, minerals, and fluids are lost when you drink, so you need to replenish. If you want to look and feel better the day after you imbibe, there's a hangover trifecta. After a night out, drink eight ounces of coconut water, take a B-complex vitamin, and eat a few strawberries for vitamin C. For the next day, bone broth with ginger is a lifesaver (and beauty-saver) thanks to collagen for skin and an abundance of minerals.

keep the fat

Not all fats are bad for you. In fact, healthy fats can keep your skin looking younger and plumper. There are many sources of good fats, such as nuts, fish, and many types of oils. Fats are also a great way to nourish the body and keep you fuller longer. I've learned a lot about health and food from nutritionist and chef Tricia Williams of Food Matters NYC, a company that delivers healthy meals and educates clients about nutritious food. I asked Tricia to share her wisdom on the best sources of good fats:

ANIMAL FATS: There is a shift happening in the health food movement to return to eating and cooking the way traditional cultures did. Cooking with schmaltz (chicken fat) and tallow (beef or mutton fat) are great ways to support the body. Chicken fat is full of oleic acid, which helps nourish the skin. Beef tallow has a high content of CLA (conjugated linoleic acid), which has been shown to reduce heart disease and the risk of cancer. It also has high levels of vitamins A and E and is a great source of omega-3s.

COCONUT OIL: Coconut oil is a great way to nourish the body. It's a medium-chain fatty acid, meaning it can take high heat in cooking without becoming unstable (unlike olive oil). This delicious oil is easily absorbed by the small intestine, delivering more energy than any other fat. It is anti-viral, antimicrobial, and has immune-boosting properties.

OMEGA-3 FATTY ACIDS: These are key to beauty from the inside out. They are anti-inflammatory, reducing inflammation under the skin's surface. They restore moisture to the skin and can help slow down the aging process. Delicious sources for omega-3s are wild salmon, avocados, walnuts, and chia seeds.

MEAT (RESPONSIBLY RAISED): Responsibly raised pasture meats are a good source of healthy fats. If you get fats from meat, choose versions that are free of antibiotics, so you get the full benefits. Williams says, "Examples of healthy meats are grass-fed lamb, bison, grass-fed beef, chicken, and duck. The meat doesn't necessarily need to be lean. Full fat in small quantities is good for you."

NUT AND SEED OILS: These oils can help you look younger. I love oils that are higher in vitamin K and E, such as almond oil, macadamia nut oil, pumpkin seed oil, and grapeseed oil.

OLIVES AND OLIVE OIL: These are rich sources of vitamins A and E, which are important skin-protecting vitamins. They help strengthen the connective tissues in the body, help improve the appearance of skin, and help protect against UV radiation.

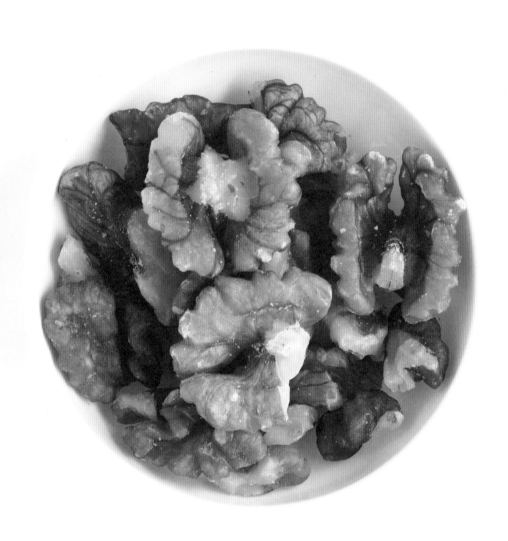

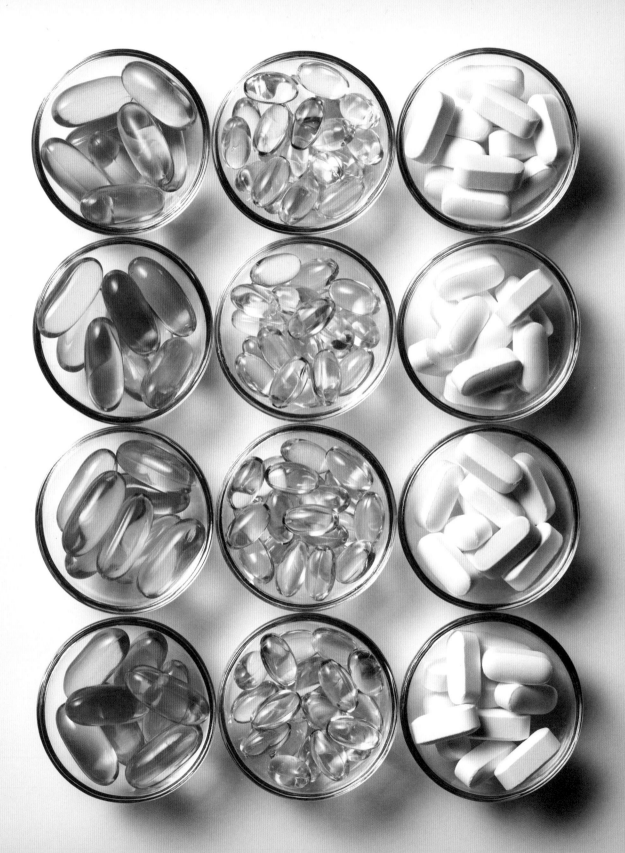

supplements

If you want a beauty boost for creating gorgeous skin and strong bones, hair, nails, and teeth, start with a healthy diet. Supplements can help, but don't expect them to do all the work or make up for bad habits. When added to a healthy diet and lifestyle, supplements can enhance your overall glow and well-being and help with a range of beauty issues, from acne to hair loss.

There are plenty of opinions out there on supplements. Some experts say they are essential and others say they are unnecessary. Navigating all of the options can get confusing. I try to keep it simple. As a baseline I take supplements for nutrients that are difficult to get from food alone (and naturally lacking in most people). I take fish oil, a probiotic, and vitamin D3. The omega-3s in the fish oil and the probiotic boost gut health, which can help to heal and prevent skin issues, increase skin elasticity, promote hair growth, and possibly even reduce the appearance of lines. Vitamin D3 is excellent for preventing cognitive decline and heart disease. For stress, a B-complex vitamin is a good addition, as B vitamins aren't stored in your body and they help with energy, mood, and brain function. For improved sleep, try magnesium, which balances the nervous system and helps you relax, and melatonin, which is a hormone linked to sleep.

Talk to your doctor or nutritionist and educate yourself before starting daily supplements. You will also need to seek professional input when you are pregnant or taking other medications. Adapt and adjust your supplement intake based on your specific health situation.

gut health

Many doctors and nutritionists believe there is a direct connection between gut health and overall health. An unhealthy gut has been linked to everything from compromised immunity, brain fog, bloating, and skin issues (which makes sense, as the skin is the largest organ in the body). "When a client has a skin issue, I always know we have to fix what's going on in the gut," says alkaline diet expert, nutritionist, and chiropractor Daryl Gioffre. Gut issues are more common than you might think thanks to antibiotics (which kill both good and bad bacteria), poor diet, and pesticides. Thankfully, getting your gut—and your skin—back on track is easier than you think. It starts with a combination of probiotics and prebiotics. Here Gioffre weighs in:

PROBIOTICS

You really are what you eat. I take it one step further and say you are what you absorb. You can eat good, healthy things, but if your digestive system is in an acidic state or an inflamed state, your body isn't able to absorb all the nutrients in the food. It creates inflammation, fungus, an overgrowth of bad bacteria, and a leaky gut. When these toxins and acids enter your bloodstream where they don't belong, your body will do anything to get them out, and one of the ways it does is through the skin. This can lead to acne, psoriasis, dermatitis, eczema, sagging and wrinkled skin, blemishes, moles, and blisters. If you have any skin issue, you need to focus on treating and healing your gut with probiotics, chlorophyll, minerals, and omega-3 fatty acids.

Pesticides, herbicides, poor nutrition, prescription drugs, industrial farming, and antibiotics all destroy the healthy bacteria in the body that is essential for good health. Most people just don't have the healthy bacteria that our bodies need, so taking a probiotic is essential. If you take a supplement twice a day, probiotics work immediately to improve the function of the digestive track. A probiotic supplement in capsule or liquid form is your best source. While some doctors recommend yogurt and kombucha, I believe they make the body more acidic and don't provide enough of the healthy bacteria needed.

Keep in mind that the number of CFUs (colony forming units) on the label of a probiotic is going to be significantly reduced when it is ingested. Due to heat and moisture in the body, there is going to be a die-off of the probiotic bacteria. Try to get a brand that has 19 or 20 billion CFUs in it. A version with live bacteria that has to be refrigerated will be your best source. The most important strains to look for are Lactobacillus acidophilus DDS-1, Lactobacillus plantarum (what our pre-agricultural ancestors' diet consisted of), Lactobacillus casei, Lactobacillus salivarius, Lactobacillus rhamnosus, and Lactobacillus brevis. It is important to alternate probiotic brands every 90 days so that you can be assured your body is getting all of the necessary strains it needs. The digestive tract responds better to variety and change.

PREBIOTICS

Prebiotics are specialized plant fibers that the body does not digest that nourish the good bacteria in your digestive tract to help it flourish. Good food sources of prebiotics include leafy green alkaline vegetables such as kale, spinach, watercress, and dandelion greens, as well as artichokes, asparagus, garlic, leeks, onions, jicama, and chicory root.

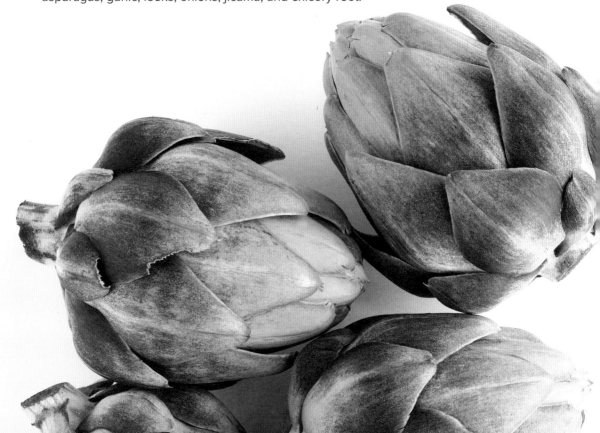

digestion and metabolism

Healthy digestion and a steady metabolism are crucial to feeling and looking great, but many women inadvertently cause their metabolisms to slow down with fad diets, starving, and binging. "I tell women you cannot starve yourself skinny, because long-term it will have the opposite effect," explains Dr. Amy Shah, who combines Eastern and Western medicine in her practice. To regulate your metabolism, Shah recommends eating three meals a day to balance your body's natural hunger signals. "Think of food as nourishment, not as something to avoid," Shah advises. To help gently shed fat and reduce inflammation without skipping meals, she suggests not eating after 7 p.m. once a week along with regularly incorporating ginger, garlic, and turmeric into your diet. Sleeping between 6 and 8 hours will also make a difference. "Sleep is the biggest shortcut to anti-aging, anti-inflammation, and better digestion," explains Dr. Shah.

vitamins for beauty

Supplements provide an additional nutrient boost that can be helpful for targeting specific concerns. "It is difficult to get all the nutrients you need for optimal nutrition from diet alone," explains Dr. Frank Lipman. A pioneer in integrative medicine, Dr. Lipman works with clients to understand how food, supplements, herbs, exercise, alternative therapies, and relaxation all work in tandem to create optimal health. Here are the vitamins he recommends. (Be sure to consult with your own doctor or nutritionist to get specific vitamins and dosages tailored to your particular needs.)

VITAMIN / SUPPLEMENT	HEALTHY SKIN	HEALTHY HAIR	STRONG NAILS	ACNE	AGING SKIN	HAIR LOSS
biotin	●	●	●			●
glutathione	●					
iron		●	●			●
manganese	●					
omega-3 fatty acids	●	●			●	●
probiotics	●			●		
silica		●				●
zinc	●	●	●	●		●
vitamin A	●			●		
B-complex vitamins		●	●			●
vitamin C	●		●			●
vitamin D	●	●				
vitamin E	●					
vitamin K	●					

beauty herbs

TWO HERBALISTS WEIGH IN

Herbs have been used for beauty for centuries. Herbalists Summer Ashley Singletary and Sarah Kate Benjamin of the Great Kosmic Kitchen are experts in the art of herbal remedies. They believe in incorporating herbs into smoothies, teas, and facial care products to reap their health and beauty benefits daily. Here are six herbs to start working into your routine.

BURDOCK
Arctium lappa
PLANT PARTS USED: Primarily root and seeds
WHAT IT DOES: Otherwise known as "gobo," burdock is a cooling, alkalizing plant rich in iron, magnesium, and manganese. It targets the liver and helps treat stagnant conditions of the blood, and it is great for clearing skin problems such as eczema, psoriasis, and acne. Use the fresh roots in soups, add them to stir-fries, pickle them, or infuse them into apple cider vinegar.

CALENDULA
Calendula officinalis
PLANT PARTS USED: Flowers
WHAT IT DOES: Oils infused with calendula flowers can be used in soothing salves and creams or applied directly on the skin to address dermatitis, psoriasis, or eczema. Calendula is also known to aid in the speedy healing of wounds. (It was used on wounded soldiers in World War I.) Try adding these vibrant beauties to salads, herbal butters, and facial steams, or create your own calendula-infused facial oil for brighter, calmer skin. This can be done by filling a jar halfway with dried calendula flowers and topping it off with almond or sesame oil. Then seal the jar and set it on a sunny windowsill for four to six weeks. Once the petals are strained out, you can use this infused oil to nourish the skin and promote a vibrant complexion.

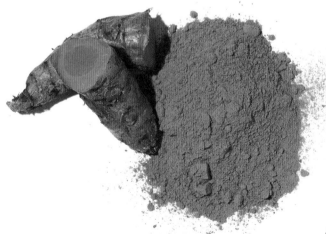

DANDELION

Taraxacum officinale

PLANT PARTS USED: Leaves and roots

WHAT IT DOES: One of the weeds most revered by herbalists, this bitter and delicious green can be eaten for various health benefits. The fresh, young, toothed leaves are high in vitamins and minerals. Add them to your favorite pesto recipe for a medicinal kick, slice them into your salad greens, lightly cook them in olive oil or butter, use them to garnish a soup, or eat them on their own with salt, pepper, lemon, and feta. The roots are often ingested for their bitter flavor, which stimulates the liver and helps with digestion. You can also use the plant's dried roots with chicory and medicinal mushrooms such as reishi, combining them with hot water as an herbal coffee substitute to support the body's natural systems of detoxification. Our favorite handcrafted blend is Reishi Roast by Farmacopia, or you can source herbs in bulk from Mountain Rose Herbs to craft your own herbal beauty blend.

———

NETTLE

Urtica dioica

PLANT PARTS USED: Leaves, seeds, and root

WHAT IT DOES: Nettle is a nourishing tonic herb that feeds the entire body. This plant is packed with vitamins and minerals including calcium, magnesium, iron, potassium, phosphorus, manganese, and vitamins C and B. Nettle helps with eczema and seasonal allergies and promotes joint health. The fresh leaves can be enjoyed as a tea or chopped and cooked as a green in frittatas, soups, or stir-fries.

RED CLOVER

Trifolium pratense

PLANT PARTS USED: Flowers

WHAT IT DOES: Red clover works to support the body's natural systems of detoxification. It is a great herb to help with chronic respiratory issues or inflammatory skin conditions such as eczema and psoriasis. This tiny purple wildflower also holds an abundance of vitamins and minerals, including calcium, magnesium, and vitamin C. Recent studies have identified isoflavones (compounds that act like estrogen in the body) in red clover that can help women with hormone imbalances and menopausal symptoms. Try making a tea of this tasty herb to sip and enjoy, or use the tea externally, as a wash or facial steam, for extra skin support.

———

TURMERIC

Curcuma longa

PLANT PARTS USED: Rhizome

WHAT IT DOES: This bitter and astringent herb has a long history of use in ancient Ayurvedic practices and is known to treat digestive disorders, skin infections, and inflammation. It increases bile production, which helps with the breakdown of fats during digestion. To use it as a skin tonic, mix turmeric powder into a warm cup of organic whole dairy milk or milk alternative (commonly called golden milk). Adding a pinch of black pepper helps activate turmeric's healing properties for skin and inflammation.

beauty food recipes

A CLEAN FOOD CHEF WEIGHS IN

It's one thing to be motivated to eat healthier, but ultimately success comes down to taste. I am a foodie—but a health foodie, always in search of delicious yet clean food. I get a lot of inspiration from food blogs and Instagram, which is where I discovered Lily Kunin, the founder of *Clean Food Dirty City.* A cook as well as a food and health coach, Lily puts together super-cool recipes that are easy to make and that combine some unexpected and delicious foods. Her photography is also gorgeous and will inspire you to get to work in the kitchen. I've been lucky enough to eat her food, and I would have her move in with me if I could. Here are some of Lily's best beauty food recipes.

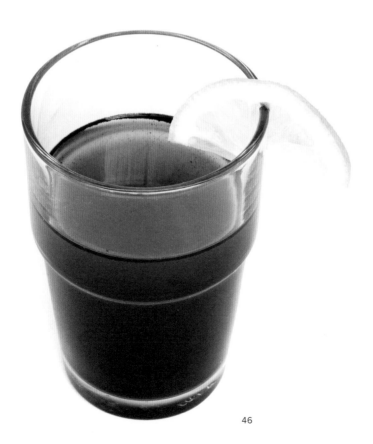

CHLORELLA MORNING TONIC

Rich with chlorophyll, chlorella is one of the greatest superfoods on the planet. High in protein and B vitamins, it is mega-detoxifying. Drink this tonic every morning for a hydrating, energizing, beauty-boosting elixir that is especially great for glowing skin.

INGREDIENTS

1 cup/240 ml filtered water
½ tsp chlorella
Splash of aloe water
Squeeze of lemon

STEPS

Stir all ingredients together and enjoy first thing in the morning.

SERVES 1

AVO DIP WITH RAINBOW VEGGIES

Both avocado and hemp hearts are chock-full of omega-3s, making this afternoon snack or appetizer a secret powerhouse. Choose a variety of fresh, colorful veggies; eating the rainbow ensures you get a variety of vitamins and minerals. You can find hemp hearts at well-stocked grocers or your local health food store.

INGREDIENTS

1 avocado, peeled and pitted
1 small zucchini, chopped
2 Tbsp hemp hearts
1 garlic clove (optional)
1 lemon, juiced
¼ cup/30 ml olive oil
Sea salt and freshly ground black pepper
Seasonal vegetables (such as red peppers, carrots, cucumbers, and radishes), sliced, for serving

STEPS

In a food processor or blender, combine the avocado, zucchini, hemp hearts, garlic (if using), lemon, and olive oil and blend until smooth. Season with salt and pepper. Serve with sliced seasonal vegetables.

SERVES 4

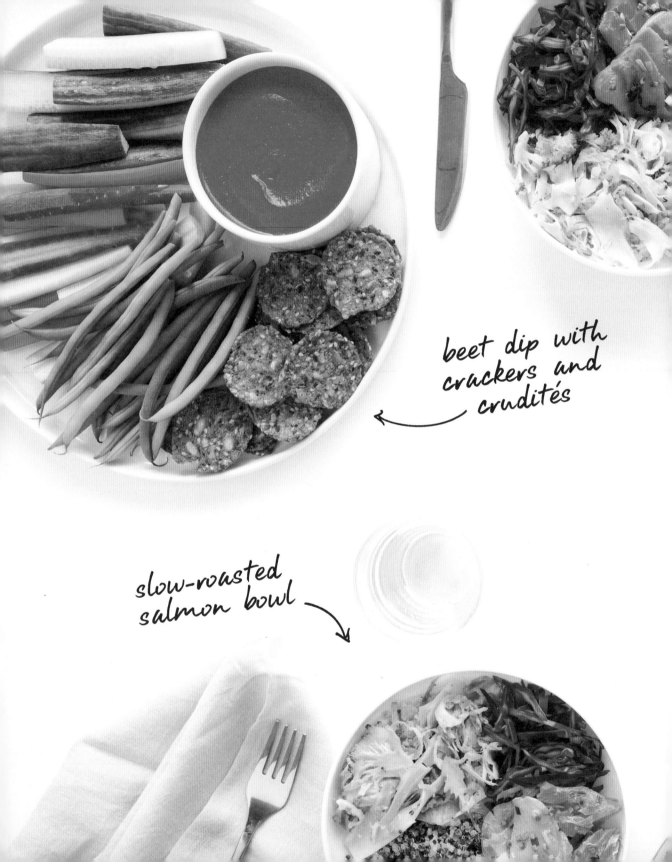

beet dip with crackers and crudités

slow-roasted salmon bowl

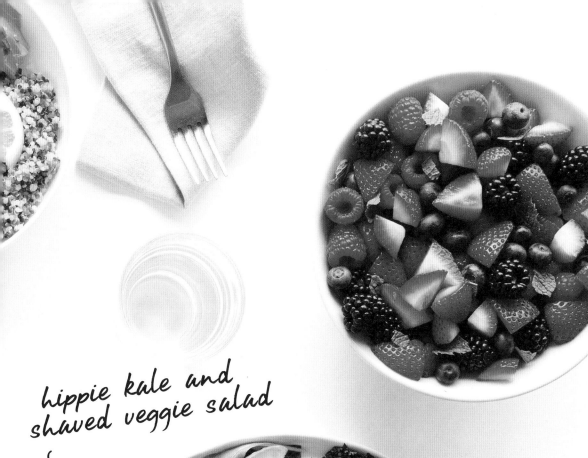

hippie kale and
shaved veggie salad

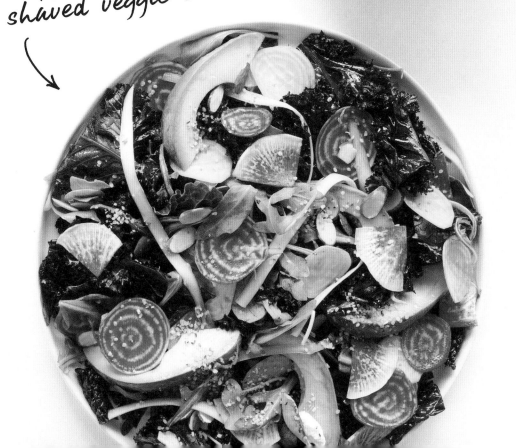

BEET DIP WITH CRACKERS AND CRUDITÉS

Beets are incredibly detoxifying and, when paired with creamy tahini, make a beautiful and delicious dip. This healthy dip is a favorite for parties and can also double as a topping for roasted vegetables.

INGREDIENTS

2 small beets
One 16-ounce/250-g can cannellini beans
  (rinsed and drained)
¼ cup/55 g tahini
3 to 4 Tbsp freshly squeezed lemon juice
2 Tbsp olive oil
Sea salt
Seasonal vegetables (such as red peppers,
  carrots, cucumbers, and radishes), sliced,
  for serving
Seed crackers, for serving

STEPS

1 Preheat the oven to 375°F/190°C. Trim and wash the beets and wrap each one tightly in foil. Bake on a baking sheet for 45 minutes to 1 hour, or until a knife pierces through them easily. Remove and let cool before peeling, then roughly chop.

2 Place the beets, beans, tahini, 2 Tbsp of the lemon juice, and a few pinches of salt into a blender or food processor. Blend until completely smooth. Drizzle in the olive oil. Season with sea salt. Taste and add more lemon juice if desired. Serve with sliced seasonal vegetables and seed crackers.

SERVES 4 TO 6

HIPPIE KALE AND SHAVED VEGGIE SALAD

The more colorful the salad, the better! It's pretty incredible that these stunning vegetables are found in nature. And they happen to be some of the most nutrient-rich foods around.

INGREDIENTS

2 Tbsp freshly squeezed lemon juice

4 Tbsp/60 ml olive oil

1 garlic clove, smashed

1 tsp raw honey

Sea salt and freshly ground black pepper

1 head of purple (or any other variety) kale, stems removed and roughly chopped

1 cup/20 g arugula

4 stalks asparagus, shaved

1 Chioggia beet, thinly sliced

1 golden beet, thinly sliced

1 watermelon radish, thinly sliced

1 avocado, peeled, pitted, and cut into ¼-inch/6-mm slices

¼ cup/25 g sliced almonds, toasted

Hemp hearts, for topping

STEPS

1 In a small bowl, combine the lemon juice, 2 Tbsp of the olive oil, the garlic, and honey and season with salt and pepper. Set aside.

2 In a medium bowl, mix the kale with a pinch of salt and drizzle in the remaining 2 Tbsp olive oil until the kale is slightly wilted and bright green. Add in the arugula, asparagus, beets, radish, avocado, and half of the almonds. Remove the garlic clove from the dressing bowl. Pour the dressing over the vegetables and toss until everything is well coated. Season with salt and pepper. Top with the hemp hearts and the rest of the almonds.

SERVES 4

SLOW-ROASTED SALMON BOWLS

Chock-full of skin-plumping healthy fats, wild salmon is one of the greatest beauty foods. This salmon stands alone as a main dish, but is also amazing when accompanied by this nutrient-rich green veggie slaw.

INGREDIENTS

1 lb/455 g wild salmon
Sea salt and freshly ground black pepper
Thyme, rosemary, and chives, for topping
1 lemon, zested and juiced
Olive oil, for topping
1 cup/60 g shredded red cabbage
2 cups/240 g cooked quinoa

Broccoli Slaw
1 shallot, minced
1 tsp Dijon mustard
1 tsp raw honey
2 Tbsp freshly squeezed lemon juice
¼ cup/60 ml olive oil
Sea salt and freshly ground black pepper
2 cups/120 g shredded broccoli
1 cup/60g shredded Brussels sprouts

STEPS

1 Preheat the oven to 250°F/120°C and line a baking sheet with parchment. Place the salmon skin-side down on the baking sheet. Top with salt, thyme, rosemary, and chives. Add some lemon zest and a drizzle of olive oil. Roast in the oven for 25 to 30 minutes, depending on the thickness of the salmon, until you can easily pierce through the fish and flake it with a fork.

2 While the fish is cooking, toss the cabbage with olive oil and lemon juice, and season with salt and pepper. Set aside.

3 In a medium bowl, combine the shallot, mustard, honey, lemon juice, olive oil, and salt and pepper. Mix well. Add the broccoli and the Brussels sprouts; make sure the vegetables are generously coated with the dressing. Add more olive oil and lemon juice as needed. Season with salt and pepper.

4 Gently flake the salmon and serve with the cabbage, quinoa, and broccoli slaw.

SERVES 4

ALL GREENS SMOOTHIE BOWL

This smoothie combines the radiance-boosting power of green fruits and veggies, including watercress, which is high in phytonutrients and vitamins K, C, and A.

INGREDIENTS

1 banana, frozen
1 pear, chopped
1 apple, chopped
¼ cup/40 g spinach
¼ cup/40 g watercress
Unsweetened almond milk, to blend
1 kiwi, chopped, for topping
Pumpkin seeds, for topping
Chopped green apple, for topping
Coconut flakes, for topping

STEPS

Combine the banana, pear, apple, spinach, and watercress in a blender and blend until smooth, adding almond milk to achieve the desired consistency. Serve in a bowl and top with the kiwi, pumpkin seeds, chopped apple, and coconut flakes.

SERVES 2 OR 3

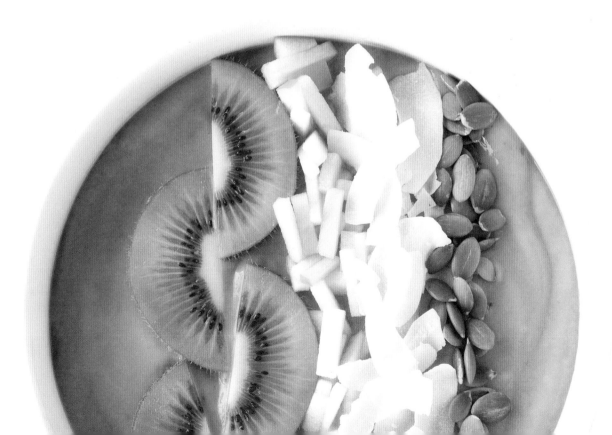

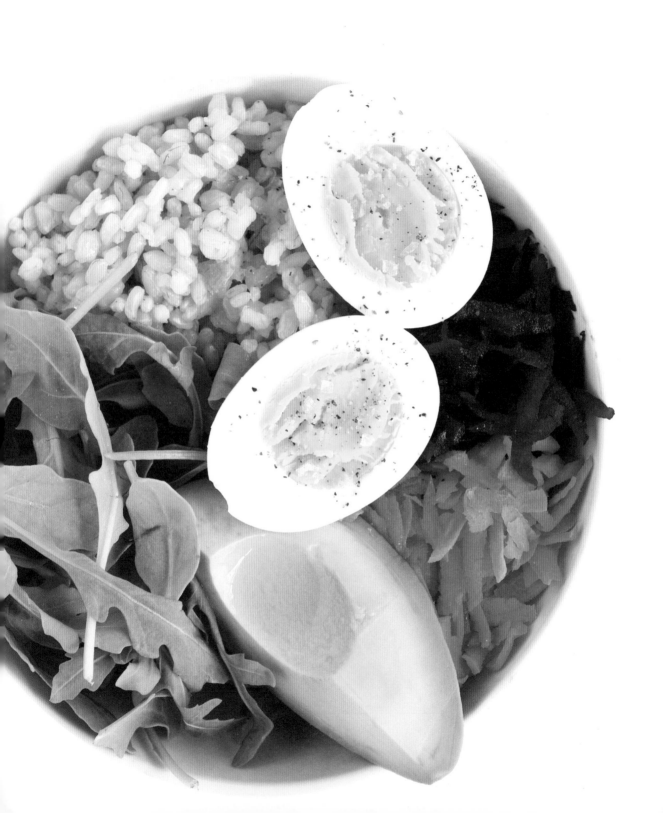

EASY MORNING BRUNCH BOWL

Start the day off right with a healthy combo of brown rice, beets, avocado, arugula, and eggs in this delicious breakfast bowl. Prep everything the evening before (minus the eggs) to make the morning a breeze.

INGREDIENTS

Miso Ginger Dressing
3 Tbsp olive oil
1 Tbsp toasted sesame oil
2 Tbsp/30 ml miso paste
1 lime, juiced
Fresh ginger, 1-inch/2.5-cm piece, chopped
Sea salt and freshly ground black pepper

1 cup/120 g cooked brown rice
1 small raw beet, grated
2 small carrots, grated
½ avocado, peeled and pitted
½ cup/10 g arugula
Drizzle of olive oil
½ lemon, juiced
Sea salt and freshly ground black pepper
2 eggs, soft- or hard-boiled

STEPS

1 To make the dressing, combine the olive oil, sesame oil, miso paste, lime juice, and ginger in a food processor and blend until smooth. Season with salt and freshly ground black pepper.

2 In a medium bowl, combine the brown rice, beet, carrots, avocado, and arugula. Drizzle with the olive oil and lemon juice, and season with salt and freshly ground black pepper. Place the eggs on top and drizzle with the miso ginger dressing. Season with salt and freshly ground pepper.

SERVES 2

BASIC BEAUTY BOWL

The ultimate beauty-food lunch combines protein, healthy fats, and veggies for a perfectly balanced bowl. Feel free to mix up the vegetables based on what's in season, and make this your go-to weekday lunch.

INGREDIENTS

Tahini Dressing
¼ cup/55 g tahini
1 to 2 Tbsp freshly squeezed lemon juice
¼ cup/60 ml warm water
Sea salt and freshly ground black pepper

1 cup/200 g cooked lentils
1 cup/120 g cooked quinoa
1 cup/120 g cubed and steamed
   sweet potato
¼ cup/40 g cherry tomatoes
4 kale leaves, cut into ¼-inch/6-mm slices
1 watermelon radish, cut into
   ⅛-inch/4-mm slices
½ avocado, peeled, pitted, and cut into
   ¼-inch/4-mm slices
Pumpkin seeds, for topping
Hemp hearts, for topping
Lemon wedge, for topping

STEPS

1 For the dressing, whisk together the tahini, lemon juice, and water in a small bowl. Season with salt and pepper.

2 Divide the lentils and quinoa between two medium bowls and add the sweet potato, tomatoes, kale, radish, and avocado. Top with tahini dressing, pumpkin seeds, hemp hearts, and a lemon wedge.

SERVES 2

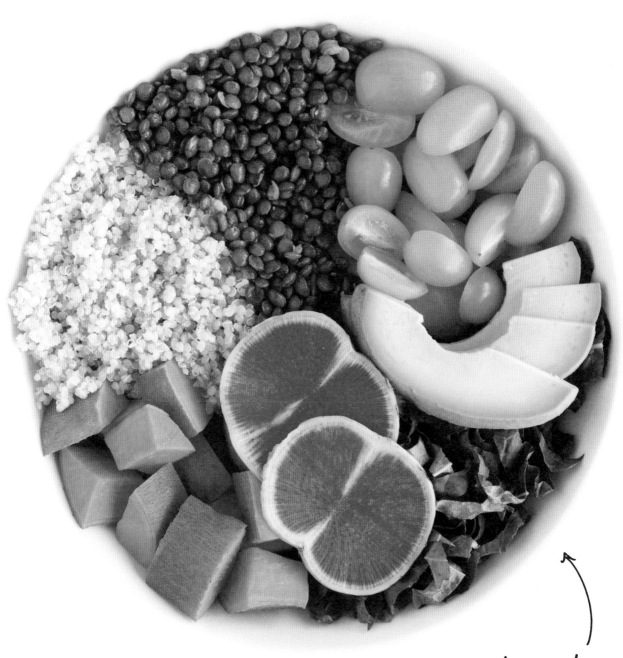

the ultimate
lunch for
glowing skin

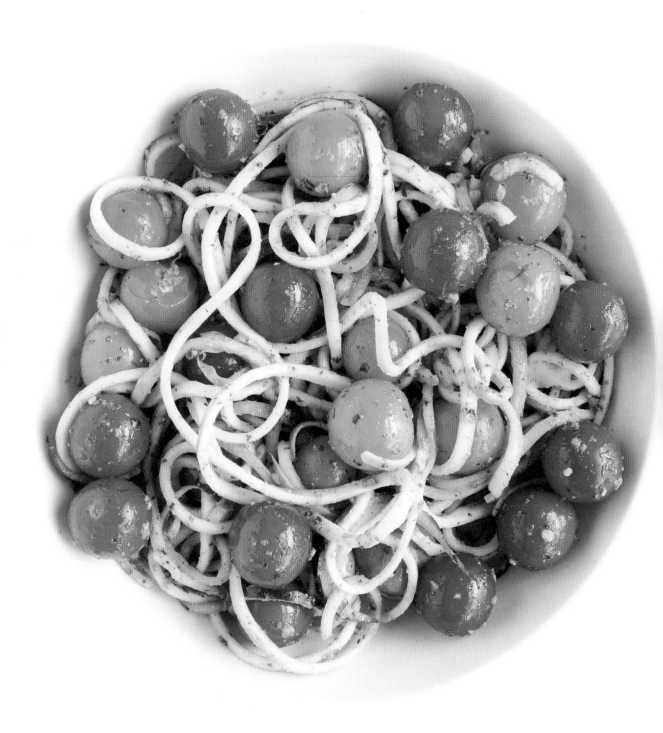

SUPER GREENS PESTO ZUCCHINI NOODLES

Pesto is a great way to sneak more greens into any dish. Made with kale and basil and mixed with zucchini noodles, pesto doubles the green goodness of this wholesome yet light meal.

INGREDIENTS

Pistachio Pesto
¼ cup/35 g pistachios, toasted
1 cup/12 g packed basil leaves
1 cup/15 g chopped Tuscan kale
½ lemon, juiced
½ tsp sea salt
¼ cup/60 ml olive oil

4 zucchini, spiralized or julienned
2 cups/320 g mixed tomatoes, diced

STEPS

1 To make the pesto, pulse the pistachios, basil, kale, lemon juice, and salt in a food processor or blender. Drizzle in the olive oil, adding more as needed for the desired consistency. Season with salt and more lemon juice.

2 Toss the vegetable "noodles" with a generous amount of pesto. Gently stir in half of the tomatoes. Top with the remaining tomatoes before serving.

SERVES 4

BLUEBERRY COCONUT CHIA PUDDING

This healthy breakfast easily doubles as a perfect afternoon snack. Chia seeds are great for digestion and high in omega-3s and will keep you feeling full and energized.

INGREDIENTS

1 cup/240 ml almond milk
½ cup/70 g blueberries
3 Tbsp chia seeds
Dash of vanilla extract
Cinnamon
Sea salt
Raw honey (optional)
Blueberries, raspberries, strawberries, or
   goji berries, for topping
Coconut flakes

STEPS

In a blender, combine the almond milk and blueberries; puree until smooth. Strain the mixture into a bowl using a fine mesh strainer or nut milk bag. Stir in the chia seeds. Add a dash of vanilla extract, and season with cinnamon, sea salt, and honey (if using) to taste. Top with blueberries, raspberries, or goji berries. Sprinkle with coconut flakes and serve.

SERVES 2

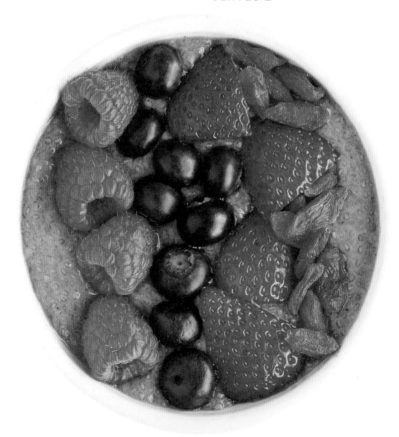

CITRUS COCO YOGURT WITH PISTACHIO BITS

The base of this satisfying breakfast or snack is coconut yogurt, which contains healthy fats and gut-restoring probiotics. Citrus adds a hydrating boost for the skin and is chock-full of vitamin C.

INGREDIENTS

1 cup/240 g coconut yogurt
2 Tbsp chopped pistachios, toasted
Assorted citrus fruits (blood oranges, navel oranges, and grapefruit), peeled and sliced

STEPS

Divide the coconut yogurt between two bowls and top with citrus and pistachios.

SERVES 2

A one-two punch of skin-loving vitamin C and gut-restoring probiotics.

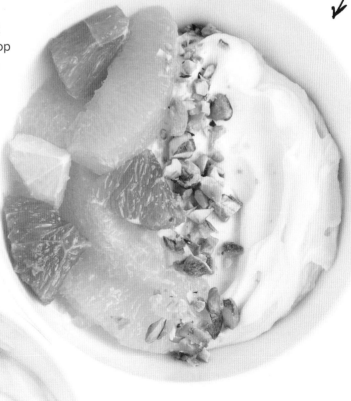

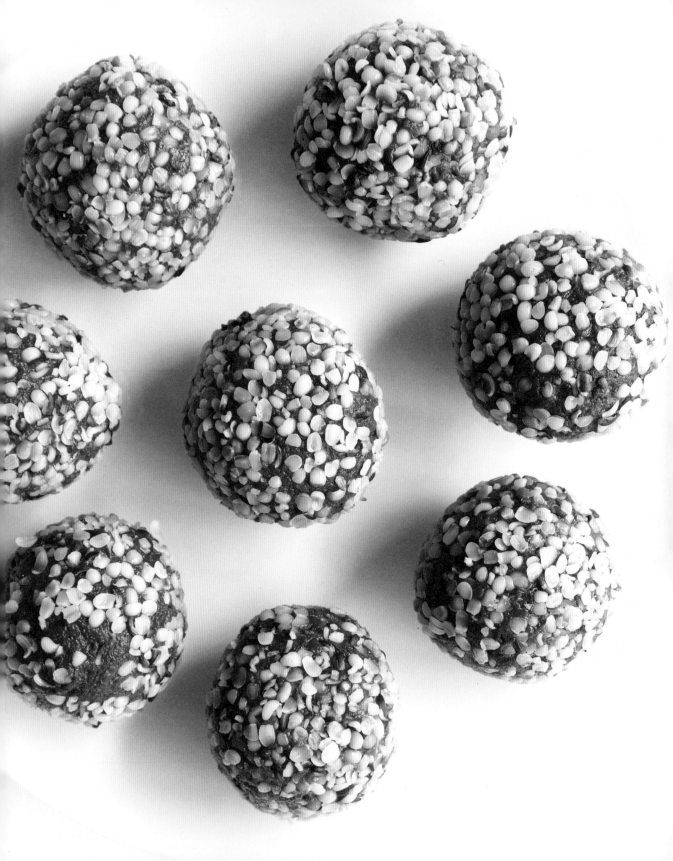

WALNUT CACAO BEAUTY BITES

This is a good-for-you indulgence with deep notes of cacao. Don't skip toasting the walnuts, as it removes the bitterness and gives these bites an irresistible espresso-like flavor.

INGREDIENTS

1 cup/120 g chopped walnuts
1 cup/150g medjool dates, pitted
¼ cup/20 g raw cacao powder
¼ tsp sea salt
¼ tsp vanilla extract
Hemp hearts, for topping

STEPS

1 Preheat the oven to 350°F/180°C. Place the walnuts on a baking sheet in a single layer. Bake for 8 to 10 minutes, checking frequently.

2 Combine the toasted walnuts, dates, cacao powder, salt, and vanilla extract in a food processor and blend until well combined, adding 1 Tbsp of warm water at a time as needed for consistency. Scoop the mixture into a medium bowl and place in the freezer for about 30 minutes.

3 Use a teaspoon to scoop out dough and then roll into balls. Coat the balls in hemp hearts and store in the freezer until ready to enjoy.

MAKES 12

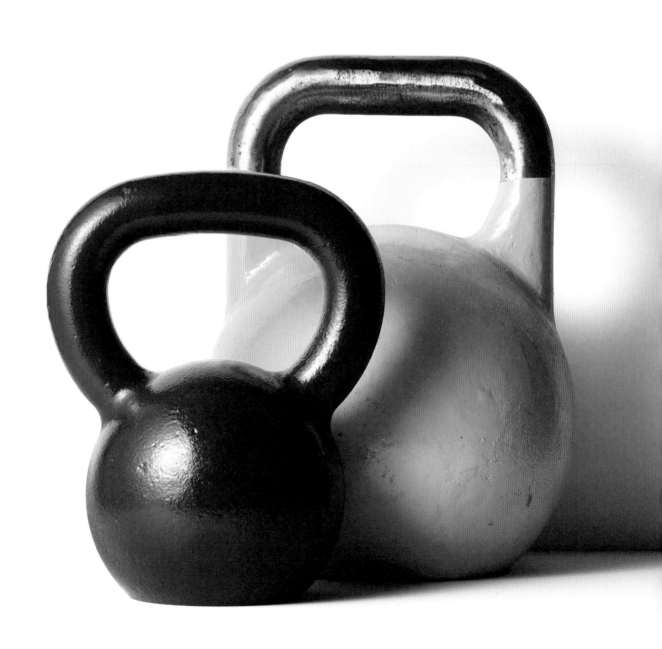

Strength

2

Strong is beautiful. It's also empowering. Being able to run a mile, lift weights, hold difficult poses, or walk 10,000-plus steps feels great. You get an incredible high from being able to accomplish something challenging. This is about more than endorphins—pushing your body transforms your attitude, how you feel about yourself, and how you look, too. It's a mood changer and stress buster. Weight drops off, you get more chiseled, and you look and feel better. Plus, there's a sense of confidence that comes with kicking ass at a sport or fitness challenge. The stronger you are, the more powerful you feel.

strong is better than skinny

I have always been obsessed with athletes. There is something incredibly inspiring about people who have that combination of determination, strength, and stamina.

Athletes have also inspired me to love and appreciate a fit body, including my own. After I had my first son (I eventually had three), my body didn't bounce back the way I had hoped. I started doing a lot of different exercises to gain muscle tone, flexibility, and energy. Of course, losing weight was part of it, but that wasn't my main goal—getting in shape was. I just want be as fit, flexible, and strong as I can be. That's when I feel my best.

A strong body comes in many shapes and sizes. It's not just that one pencil-thin look that you see on the runway. It celebrates muscles and curves, not just skinniness. Fitness is all about feeling great in your body.

BREAK A SWEAT

If you make exercise a regular part of your life, no matter how old you are, you will never regret it. Schedule it in your calendar like a meeting. For me, exercise isn't about what to do but when to do it. Every week, I fit several workouts into my ever-changing schedule. I do at least two weekly strength and conditioning workouts, aiming for three. I like to try new workouts when I can. I've gotten hooked on everything from yoga to spinning to boot camp. I love the mental and physical challenge that comes with pushing myself, and I like to break a sweat for at least 30 minutes at a time. I also walk often throughout the day, aiming for 12,000 steps. Vacations for me are full-on fitness jaunts. My husband and I put on our sneakers and walk. We explore the city, eat local, and walk everywhere. It's all about consistency. You can do the toughest workout, but if you do it infrequently, it won't make any difference.

CHANGE IT UP

When you do the same workout over and over, your body gets used to it and it stops being as effective. Repeating the same moves each day can also get boring. And if you're bored, you may not be motivated to keep working out.

I've found that the key is mixing it up. This might mean trying a new class, taking a new route on a run, or working with a new trainer. It's always good to do something different, and you just might love the new activity.

Changing goals and workouts can be about more than just working different muscles. Trying new things is also mentally stimulating; it breaks us out of our rut and routine.

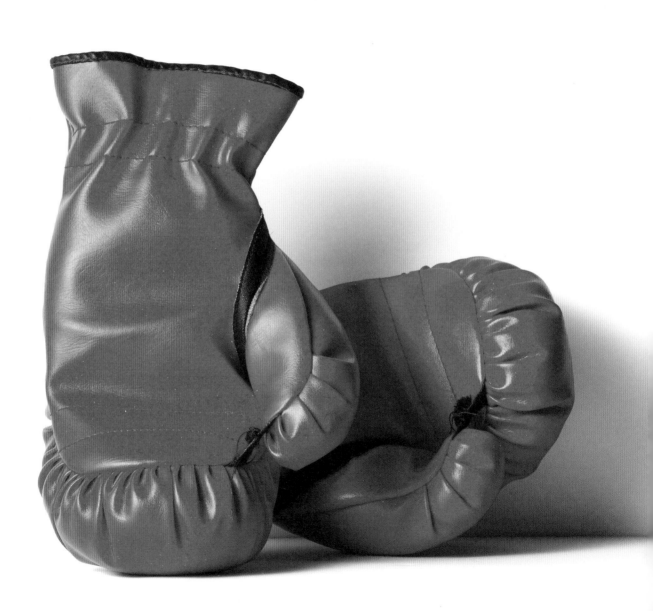

workout guide

If you want to get in shape, you've never had more options. From low-impact exercises such as walking and barre, to power classes like HIIT, to more interactive and social options such as spinning or hip-hop, you'll never get bored. Here are some of my favorite workouts.

WALKING

WHO IT'S BEST FOR: "There are no barriers to entry, so anyone can take up walking," says trainer and nutritionist Harley Pasternak. "There's no skill requirement, no equipment required. Men, women, old, and young, everyone can benefit from walking."

WHAT IT DOES: Walking is a low-impact way to get in some cardio and stay fit. According to Pasternak, walking 10,000 steps a day is good for general health, and if you walk 12,000 steps or more a day, it will help with weight loss if you are consistent.

WHY IT'S GREAT: "Walking is a great exercise option because you can weave it into your daily routine and you don't have to set time aside," explains Pasternak. "You can walk to lunch [or] take calls while walking. If you want to spend time with a friend, you can go on a walk together. A fitness tracker will help keep you motivated. For general health, you should walk 10,000 steps a day, seven days a week."

INVESTMENT: None—just comfortable walking shoes that provide enough support.

RUNNING

WHO IT'S BEST FOR: Anyone looking for a strong cardio workout that they can do pretty much anywhere, anytime, and on a budget.

WHAT IT DOES: Running is great for burning calories, melting fat, and losing weight. It targets many parts of the body: legs, glutes, core, and heart.

WHY IT'S GREAT: "There is a meditative, spiritual component to running, connecting mind and body. There isn't any sport that I have done that equates to that euphoric chemical release that your body experiences when you run," says fitness trainer David Kirsch.

INVESTMENT: Minimal. All you really need is a good pair of running shoes (these are nonnegotiable—worn-out shoes can lead to injury) and a sports bra. Once you start running longer distances, you may want to invest in clothes that feature special fabric to wick the sweat off your body. You may need seasonal clothing, too, depending on your climate. Races are a great way to stay motivated, and they generally require entry fees.

BIKING

WHO IT'S BEST FOR: Biking is a sport that can work for a variety of fitness levels because you control the pace and exertion and can coast when you want to rest. Biking is popular among all age groups in many countries around the world.

WHAT IT DOES: Works your legs, thighs, glutes, lower back, and core.

WHY IT'S GREAT: "It's good for your body, good for your psyche, good for your muscles," says Kirsch.

INVESTMENT: Moderate to high depending on the cost of your bike (there is a wide range for both mountain and road bikes) and how much fancy gear you want to add. Once you have a bike, all you really need is a helmet, but, like all sports, you can add on more gear as you improve—everything from gloves to special biking outfits complete with crotch padding. How much extra you want to invest after the bike and helmet is up to you.

FREE WEIGHTS

WHAT IT IS: Using free weights such as dumbbells, barbells, or kettlebells in repetitive movements.

WHO IT'S BEST FOR: Anyone looking for more tone and strength.

WHAT IT DOES: Depending on how much you lift, how you train, and how often you do it, weights can be used to bulk up or simply tone. It's also the perfect supplement for cardio workouts, targeting muscles in ways that cardio alone cannot.

WHY IT'S GREAT: "Research shows that those on a combination of cardio and resistance (versus just a cardio) regimen have results that are exponentially more significant and a lot more permanent," explains Pasternak. "Weight training increases bone density and muscle mass. It also has a positive impact on boosting hormones that normally decrease with age."

INVESTMENT: Minimum to moderate. Invest in a couple of sets of free weights (5 and 10 pounds would be a good start) and buy a book or download an app to get started. If you work with a trainer, that's a bigger investment, but it means your workouts will be tailored to your body type and ability.

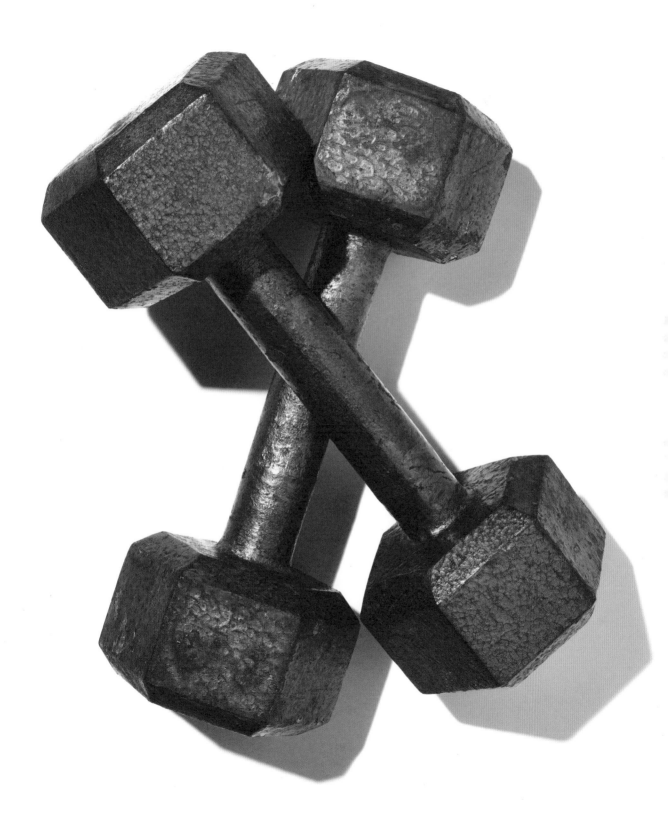

SUSPENSION TRAINING

WHAT IT IS: Performing repetitive resistance exercises using your body weight and TRX suspension straps that can hook to a wall or door.

WHO IT'S BEST FOR: Ideal for someone who wants to get toned and tight without spending a lot of money. The strengthening exercises can be done at any age.

WHAT IT DOES: Suspension training helps with balance and flexibility, tightens the core, and tones targeted muscles. "It is a good form of resistance exercise to complement other forms. The bands are a lot more cost-effective and space-effective than an entire set of dumbbells. It's one type of equipment that has the versatility to allow you to train a few body parts very well," explains Pasternak.

WHY IT'S GREAT: "Everyone should be working suspension exercises into their workout routine," says Pasternak. "They increase muscle tissue and boost your metabolism."

INVESTMENT: Minimal to moderate. The suspension bands are the only equipment needed. You can download an app or buy an instructional book for a small investment. Classes or private instruction will cost more.

MARTIAL ARTS

WHAT IT IS: Self-defense and combat practices such as karate, judo, and tae kwon do.

WHO IT'S BEST FOR: Someone who wants to learn self-defense and combat in addition to getting in shape. Ideal for someone who likes learning, setting and achieving goals, and being in a class setting. However, you need to make a commitment to the sport, as it can take time to climb the ranks.

WHAT IT DOES: Incorporates a mix of stability, balance, and high-intensity moves with little to no equipment for an excellent full-body workout. Plus, you can learn to take down a mugger.

WHY IT'S GREAT: "With martial arts, you get more than just a workout—you're learning, and there is a lot of focus on respect and integrity. It gives you goals to work toward, both physical and mental," says trainer Ashley Wilking.

INVESTMENT: Moderate. You'll need to pay for classes and purchase a uniform.

HIIT TRAINING

WHAT IT IS: HIIT stands for "high intensity interval training," which features short bursts of high-intensity workouts followed by brief periods of rest. The moves are a mix of cardio, weights, and resistance done at high speed and exertion.

WHO IT'S BEST FOR: People who are already in good physical and mental shape and want maximum results in a short time period. A great option for the time-crunched. Not recommended for anyone just starting to exercise.

WHAT IT DOES: HIIT tones your entire body from head to toe. It burns a lot of calories and boosts metabolism in a short period of time.

WHY IT'S GREAT: "HIIT has fabulous results because it creates custom circuit workouts with moves such as burpees, push-ups, lunges, and squat jumps with bursts of cardio on the treadmill or rowing machine. You see results very fast when doing these high-intensity workouts on a regular basis," explains Kirsch. "Brides love it!"

INVESTMENT: Moderate to high, depending on where you take the class.

CARDIO DANCE

WHAT IT IS: From hip-hop to Zumba, fast-paced dance classes provide an amazing cardio workout that doesn't feel like exercise.

WHO IT'S BEST FOR: Someone who wants her workouts to be fun, high-energy, and interactive. Some dance experience helps, but it is definitely not required.

WHAT IT DOES: Helps you sweat, lose weight, and burn calories.

WHY IT'S GREAT: "These classes have great energy, and people have the benefit of enjoying themselves while they work out," says Wilking. "Plus the music can be really fun."

INVESTMENT: Minimal to moderate depending on if you take classes or use DVDs. Many gym memberships come with free Zumba classes.

Get strong, feel powerful, have fun— there are so many reasons to work out.

PILATES

WHAT IT IS: Pilates actually started as a method of physical therapy. It is centered in core exercises done lying down with machines or on a mat. Unlike yoga, which is about holding poses, Pilates involves repetitive movements that target specific muscles, with a focus on gaining core strength.

WHO IT'S BEST FOR: Pilates is a good option for someone who doesn't want to do a high-intensity workout but wants to create a strong core. If you have injuries or are recovering from an injury, Pilates can be a good complement to a resistance program. For weight loss and toning, combine your Pilates practice with cardio.

WHAT IT DOES: Pilates will lengthen and strengthen. It creates long and lean muscles and strong posture.

WHY IT'S GREAT: "Pilates works all the muscles you forgot you had," explains Wilking. "It also fights against bad posture. In a world spent looking down at a digital screen, it's incredibly important to strengthen the muscles that support our spine, and Pilates does this beautifully."

INVESTMENT: Moderate to high. The least expensive option would be to invest in Pilates apps. Pilates mat classes are the next level, and classes with reformer machines are the most expensive, as they require a one-on-one session with an instructor.

SPINNING

WHAT IT IS: An indoor cycling class that focuses on high-intensity interval training, occasionally combined with weights.

WHO IT'S BEST FOR: People who love biking but want the motivation of a class setting and are looking for total-body conditioning, or those who don't want all the gear required for outdoor biking. A great option for high-intensity cardio workouts.

WHAT IT DOES: The high-intensity cardio class is good for burning calories and losing weight. The biking part targets the lower half of your body, while classes like SoulCycle also combine weights to make it a full-body workout.

WHY IT'S GREAT: "Spinning is great for someone looking to maximize cardio and calorie burn in a short period of time while also focusing on endurance training," says Wilking. "With less impact on the joints and the ability to individually manage resistance, spinning is appealing to users new to working out who want to challenge themselves without feeling left behind."

INVESTMENT: Moderate to high. Whether you buy a stationary bike to use at home or pay for classes, spinning is an investment.

HOW TO STAY MOTIVATED

To stay fit you need to be consistent. While resting is key occasionally, moving on most days is even more important. Here are three things that keep me moving:

FITNESS TRACKERS: I started wearing a fitness band a couple of years ago and I haven't stopped. Especially when you work in an office and could easily sit for hours, knowing how much you are moving in a day is important. To get my extra steps in, I will take a few breaks to walk around the block, make calls while I am walking, or use the stairs instead of the elevator. Every step counts.

APPS: From Skyfit (which walks you through hundreds of routines for treadmill, elliptical, outdoor running, yoga, and cycling fitness) to Nike+ Running (for tracking distance and pace), there are so many apps to get you moving. What's awesome about apps is that they are inexpensive or free and you don't need to spend additional money on a trainer, gym membership, or class. You can also track progress, set goals, and even compete with friends, all of which are great motivators.

FRIENDS: At six in the morning when you want to sleep in, it's helpful to know that you have someone waiting to take a class or go on a run or walk with you. Working out with friends not only makes it more fun but keeps you accountable, too.

TAKING A BREAK

As much as I love to set goals, keep moving, and stay fit, there are times when hitting the pause button is essential. Getting worn out, exhausted, and injured are the hazards of pushing yourself too hard and too much. Listen to your body. There are times when you are feeling tired and a workout is just what you need to get your energy back up. There are other times when your body might be worn out and you just need to chill and let your muscles and mind recover and recharge. If you are a type-A person like I am, understanding that resting is just as important as moving can take a minute to sink in. However, knowing when to stop is the key to staying strong. If you feel like your muscles are fatigued and really sore, or if you are exhausted after a busy time and an extra hour of sleep is desperately needed, respect what your body and mind are telling you.

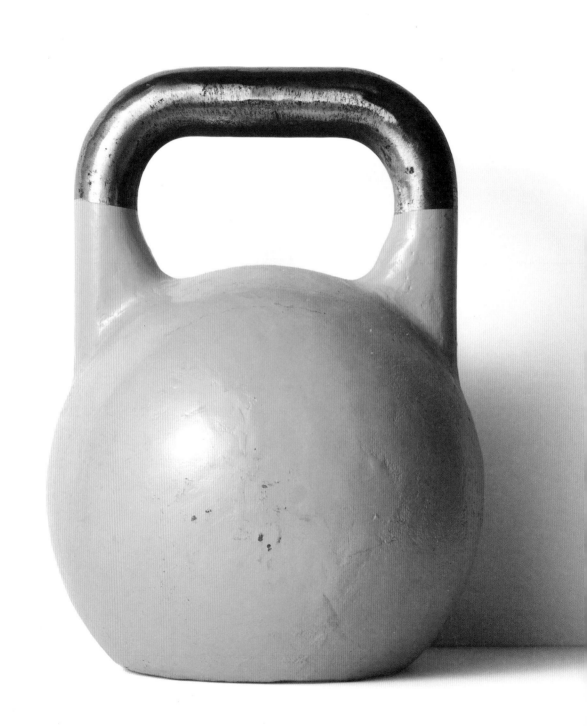

BARRE

WHAT IT IS: A total-body workout centered around core strength using a ballet barre and light free weights.

WHO IT'S BEST FOR: Barre workouts are great for those who like a challenge but don't want the intensity of a CrossFit or HIIT class. If you're looking for improved flexibility and muscle definition, this is a great option.

WHAT IT DOES: This workout improves your posture, lengthening and strengthening the body.

WHY IT'S GREAT: "Barre is a gentle and elegant workout that uses some ballet moves, but it's also extremely challenging," says Wilking. "People think it seems easy, but they walk out dazed by how tough it was."

INVESTMENT: Moderate to high. Barre classes are taught at boutique barre studios and can be pricey.

BOOT CAMP/CROSSFIT

WHAT IT IS: A workout combining strong weights with intense cardio. These classes are goal-oriented, with a number of obstacles you have to tackle.

WHO IT'S BEST FOR: Someone who likes a class that is intense, challenging, and community-based. Also those who want to set and achieve fitness goals. These classes are best for people who are physically prepared for a high-energy workout that requires both strength and endurance.

WHAT IT DOES: The main focus is on creating power and strength. You are powerlifting to gain strength and muscle mass and pairing that with plyometric moves, which combine lengthening muscle moves with shortening muscle moves for more powerful muscles.

WHY IT'S GREAT: "CrossFit involves skill-development workouts that require heavy lifting, power, and explosive movements, leaving users empowered and motivated after completing a workout or lifting a weight they never thought possible," Wilking explains.

INVESTMENT: Moderate to high. With obstacle courses, climbing walls, and drill sergeant instructors, these workouts require a specially equipped gym. Some gyms require monthly fees while others are pay-as-you-go, which can add up if you go often.

yoga

I love the mind/body connection that comes with yoga. If you want to feel and be more powerful and fit, there are poses to help you get there. If you want to be more centered, calm, and relaxed, there are poses for that, too. Kelly Stackhouse, who is based in Telluride, Colorado, is one of the best yoga teachers I know. Here she shares a series of poses designed to strengthen and a series to help you relax.

Yoga is good for everyone, regardless of fitness level, body type, or age. You can find a practice that works best for you, whether you want to improve flexibility and find deep relaxation or work up a sweat and increase your heart rate and improve your strength. Two of my preferred yoga practices are hatha, which focuses on slow movements and breath, and vinyasa, which is a vigorous flow of poses and involves holding positions for longer periods of time.

ALIGNMENT AND BREATHING

Breathing is very important for proper posture and muscle function, as well as whole body relaxation. Most people think good posture is "shoulders down and back," but this actually does more harm than good. Instead, people should focus on a long and full exhale to get their ribs down in the front and turn their abdominals on. This will put their abs in the proper position to control their spine, instead of making their backs do all the work.

Try this exercise recommended by conditioning coach Cory Plofker (who also happens to be my son):

Lie on your back with your feet flat on a wall and hips and knees at 90-degree angles. Lift your tailbone slightly off the ground while keeping your lower back flat. Inhale and then exhale slowly and fully as your ribs lower in the front. Release all the air. Repeat three sets of five breaths.

strengthening pose series

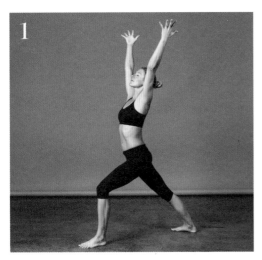

WARRIOR I/*virabhadrasana I*

This is a great warm-up pose. It gently opens the hips, chest, and lungs for better circulation and respiration.

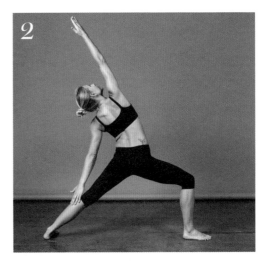

REVERSE WARRIOR/
viparita virabhadrasana

This standing pose strengthens leg muscles while lengthening through the ribs from waist to shoulders.

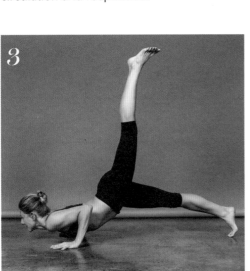

ONE-LEGGED CHATURANGA

This pose helps to develop core stability, which prepares the practitioner for inversions and arm balances.

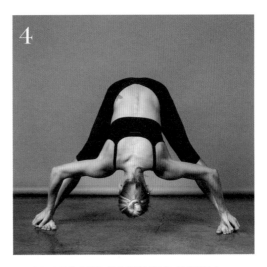

WIDE-LEGGED FORWARD BEND/
prasarita padottanasana

Coming into inversions lowers the blood pressure and calms the mind.

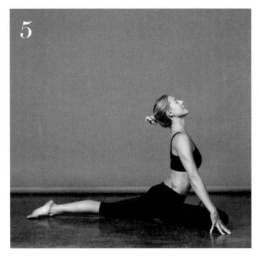

PIGEON POSE/
eka pada rajakapotasana

Pigeon pose helps release negativity and trauma through the opening of the hips.

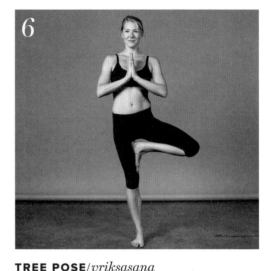

TREE POSE/*vriksasana*

The perfect pose for strengthening the core and legs while also focusing on improving balance and building stability muscles.

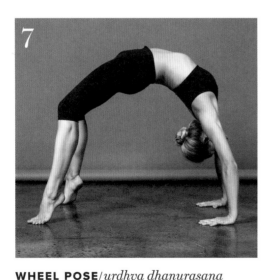

WHEEL POSE/*urdhva dhanurasana*

This heart-opening pose strengthens the arms and legs and stimulates the front line of the body.

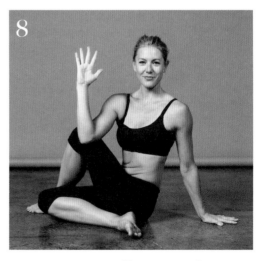

SEATED TWIST/*ardha matsyendrasana*

Twists stimulate digestion and rid the body of toxins. They help keep our spine flexible and release tension stored in the back.

relaxation pose series

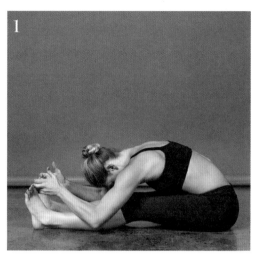

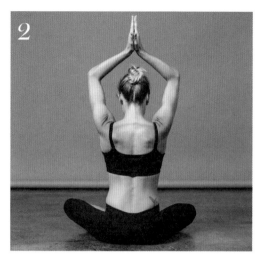

SEATED FORWARD FOLD/
paschimottanasana

This pose works deeply to open up the hamstrings and back body. It also has a strong element of surrender and release.

SEATED PRAYER TO THE SOURCE/ HIGHER SELF

This seated meditation with hands in the *namaste mudra* position focuses on love and gratitude.

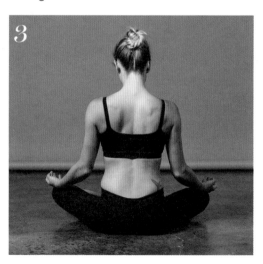

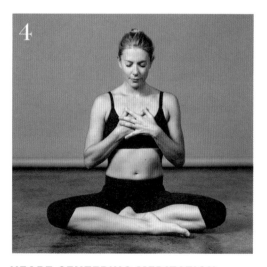

SEATED MEDITATION

With closed eyes, this pose focuses on breathing and finding the quiet and calm inside.

HEART-CENTERING MEDITATION

A focus on the heart chakra, the center of love and compassion, allows us to align the head and heart together.

power foods

A HEALTH FOOD GURU WEIGHS IN

To fuel your workouts you need good sources of energy. Protein helps you increase your metabolism, burn calories, and build muscle, while fruits and vegetables provide a nutrient boost. Shom Chowdhury, the founder of one of my favorite healthy food sources, Indie Fresh, is as passionate about fitness as he is about making healthy food delicious. These are his top power food picks:

PRE-WORKOUT FUEL: "My go-to is granola, banana, and almond milk. Bananas have a ton of potassium and digestible carbs. You can't be scared of the 'C' word—you *must* have enough energy to make any workout worthwhile and healthy," says Chowdhury. "Granola and almond milk are packed with protein, but unlike protein powders, they burn quickly and don't leave you feeling heavy and, more importantly, don't take a lot of energy to digest. Basically this is a great snack that converts to energy. Don't have enough time to grab everything? Go with the banana; it works every time."

BISON: With half the total fat of beef, bison is my top source of protein. It also has tons of B vitamins, which help with testosterone production and energy.

SALMON: One of the tastiest fish available, salmon is rich in protein, omega-3s, and amino acids. It's a great source of lean protein that helps with muscle and tissue development. Perfect for pre-workout and workout recovery.

BLACK BEANS: These are an off-the-charts source of protein and fiber, and a great way for vegans and vegetarians to get protein.

CAULIFLOWER: This is a great natural, vegan metabolism-booster and is filling, too.

BLUEBERRIES: Dark berries are great for mental focus and memory retention. I like them in pre-/post-workout smoothies, where they act as a low-calorie sweetener. They are full of antioxidants and are a great source of vitamin C.

CHERRIES: Cherries help with muscle inflammation post-workout. Their effects are similar to ginger but the taste is less harsh.

MATCHA: Think of it as a coffee sub-stitute. Drink it in the morning, and the effects last all day. Matcha is a highly concentrated green tea in powder form that provides enhanced focus and sustained energy without the crash that comes from caffeine. It also helps with detoxification.

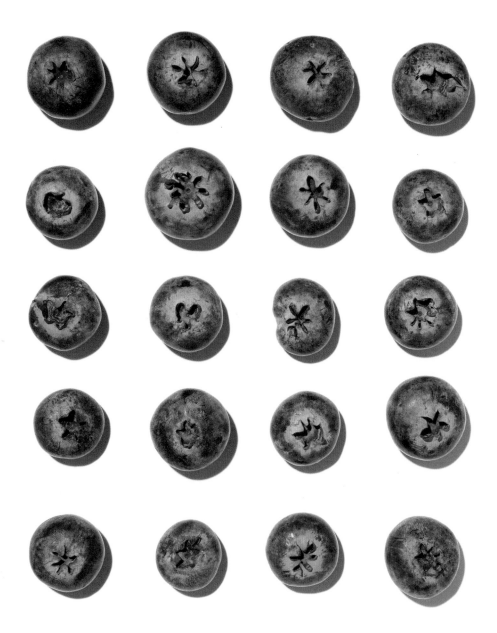

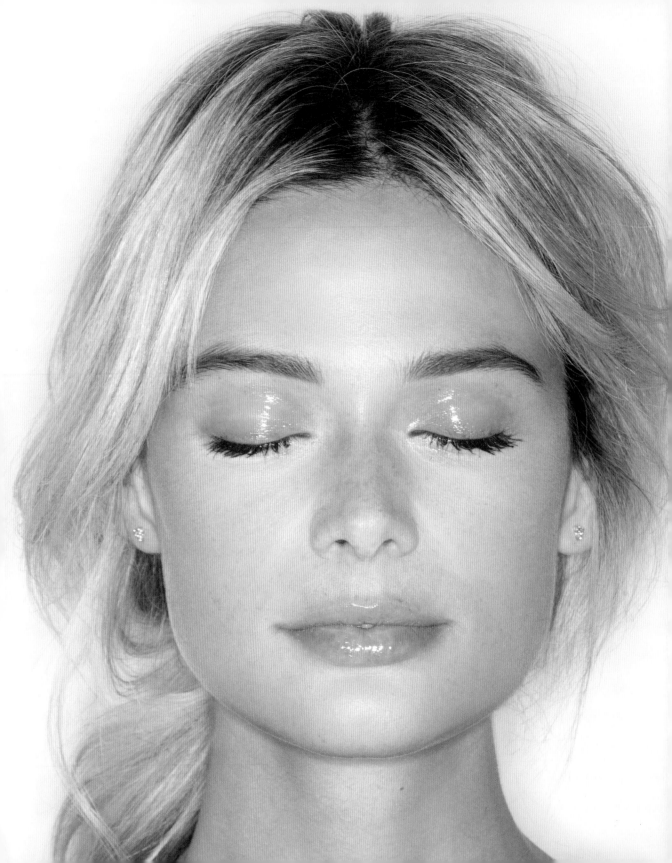

Be
Zen

*T*here is a direct link between stress and beauty. Stress shows up on your face, in your eyes, on your hair, and on your skin in a whole host of issues, from acne to dark circles. "Stress affects beauty by causing the cells in the body to divide more frequently. This affects the cellular lifespan and leads to accelerated aging and disease," explains Jeff Lally, D.C.

Experts are just beginning to understand the link between the stress hormone cortisol and how it affects you from the inside out. Everybody has it, but how you manage and process cortisol makes all the difference in how it manifests in your body and appearance. To manage stress, we need to restore our body and our mind. That means getting enough sleep (experts recommend around eight hours per night) or taking a day off from kicking ass at the gym to let muscles re-energize. It also means turning off devices occasionally—the blue light and radiation can mess with sleep cycles and increase stress levels. It's also important to quiet the mind, whether through deep breathing, a yoga class, or meditation.

For some people, taking a break sounds like heaven. For others (like me) it can be a challenge because in my mind taking a break means I am not getting something accomplished. But getting "over-everythinged"— over-stressed, over-tired, over-worked—never ends well. Some things that work for me include taking an Epsom salt bath, getting a massage, reading a book, using essential oils, or maybe turning on the TV and watching a mindless show. It's all about recharging. Taking time to restore will ultimately make you more energized and productive.

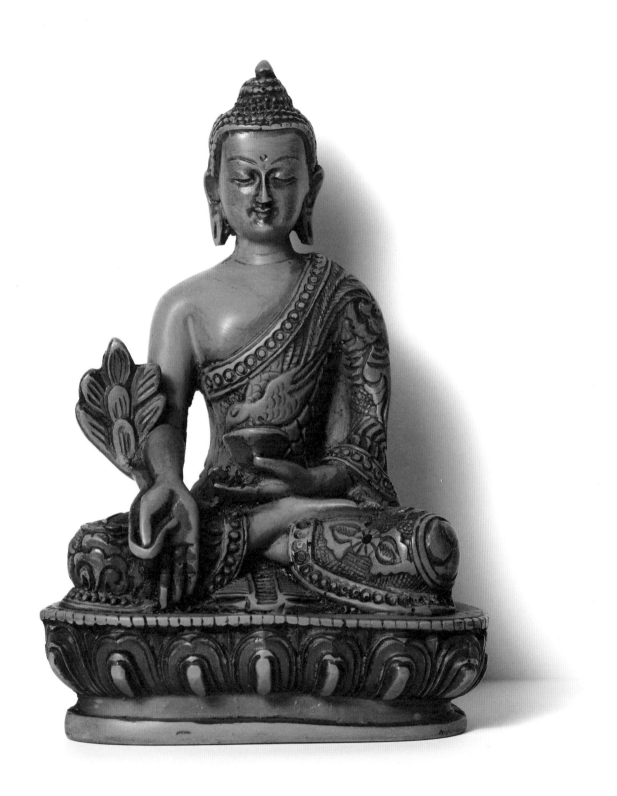

meditation:
the five-minute recharge

Whether you practice for five or forty minutes a day, there are countless benefits to meditating. Studies have shown that meditation reduces stress, lowers blood pressure, and can boost concentration. "Meditation changes the way you relate to stress. Things that used to cause you stress don't, which helps prevent stress-related illnesses such as diabetes, obesity, addiction, and heart diseases," says meditation teacher Charlie Knoles. "The top benefit is to feel happier." Who can argue with that?

While the long-term benefits of meditation are inarguable, it can help in the short term as a quick way to recharge without taking a nap. Studies have shown meditation can sometimes be more restful than sleep. Even better, you can do it for as little as five minutes a day and still see benefits. There are many different types of meditation, from simple breathwork to using a mantra. Find the best one for you.

TURN BACK THE CLOCK

There are many ways people try to slow down the clock—with creams, exercise, or dermatologist treatments. Most don't think of meditation. But studies have shown that there is a reversal of cellular aging that happens in the bodies of meditators. From the inside, your DNA repairs itself and renews cells. It may or may not affect the external markers of aging such as wrinkles or gray hair, but blood pressure, vision, hearing, and skin elasticity show a younger biological age in meditators than non-meditators. It's hard to think of a reason not to try meditation, given its relaxation benefits and anti-aging properties.

TRANSCENDENTAL

To learn this type of meditation you will have to take a workshop or meet with a meditation teacher who will give you a mantra—a sound, a word, or a series of words that will enhance your concentration. When your meditation session starts, you sit in a comfortable position, close your eyes, and simply repeat the mantra in your head to get into a relaxed state. "This type of meditation is geared toward achieving transcendence," says Knoles. "Ideally, you should practice twenty minutes a day, twice a day." Knoles says this is one of the most powerful versions of meditation and can help people de-stress almost instantly.

GUIDED

From creative visualization to hypnosis to a guided session, this meditation involves having someone help lead you into a mellow state. You can go to a class (good if you have trouble staying focused on your own) or download a free app like Insight Timer to help guide you. "It's using concentration and calm focus to achieve a different state of mind," says Knoles.

BREATHING

"This is simply closing your eyes and focusing on your breathing, not controlling it, but just being aware and bringing your concentration back to your breath when your mind wanders," explains Knoles. "It uses your breath as a tool to bring yourself back to the present moment; it's a form of practicing mindfulness." Knoles says you can benefit from as little as five minutes a day. "After about three months you'll experience measurable decreases in stress levels."

ACTIVE BREATHWORK

Some forms of meditation can get you focused and energized. "This type of practice is when you utilize control of your breath to distribute energy throughout the body to change your mindset and energize the body," explains Knoles. "Kundalini yoga and chi breathing are popular forms of active breathwork. Even athletes use these techniques before working out or competing to get their bodies and minds hyped up."

1-2-3 breathe

A MEDITATION TEACHER WEIGHS IN

Breathwork is a form of meditation, but it can also be used on its own. "Controlling your breath is the fastest way to get your mind under control," says Jen Kluczkowski, CEO of Mindfresh, a company that teaches breathwork, meditation, and mindfulness to office workers. "If your mind is whirling, you can't just tell your mind to calm down—it doesn't really work," she says. When we experience stress, breathing becomes very shallow and rapid, and the brain doesn't get all the oxygen it needs. Blood pressure and heart rate increase. Changing breathing patterns, even for just a few minutes, can help relieve these stress symptoms.

To recharge during a busy day, relax in a stressful moment, or increase productivity, Kluczkowski recommends three simple breathing exercises.

REBOOT AND FOCUS

It's amazing what simply taking a deep breath can do. If you are feeling overwhelmed at work or home and just want to reboot, try this easy exercise.

1. Breathe in deeply for a count of four.
2. Exhale for a count of four.
3. Repeat 10 times.

Bring your attention into the chest and back of the shoulders. Your first few breaths may be shallow and only engage the top front side of the chest. As your breath deepens and regulates, you will notice it expands down into the lower belly and back. "No one around you even has to know you are doing it," says Kluczkowski. "After this exercise, you'll find you have clarity and perspective that you didn't have a few minutes before."

BALANCE AND PRODUCTIVITY

"Many of us take in more breath through one nostril, which can lead to a feeling of imbalance in body and mind. The alternate nostril breathing technique allows for an even intake of air through both nostrils, creating an overall sense of equanimity after a few rounds," explains Kluczkowski.

1. Flip your right palm to face up, then pull the pointer and middle finger to the base of the thumb. Bring your right hand toward your face and plug your right nostril with your right thumb.

2. Inhale through the left nostril to the count of four, then plug the left nostril with right ring and pinky finger as you exhale out through the right nostril to the count of four.

3. Inhale through the right nostril for four, then plug the right nostril with the thumb and exhale through the left nostril for a count of four.

This completes one breath cycle. Do this for three minutes or 10 to 12 cycles.

CALM ANXIETY

To quickly calm down when you feel a surge of emotion such as stress or anger, try this:

1. Inhale for a count of three.

2. Exhale for a count of four.

3. Repeat 10 times.

The slightly longer exhale calms you quickly. Continue until you feel more relaxed.

mood changer: aromatherapy

AN AROMATHERAPIST WEIGHS IN

Aromatherapy is the practice of harnessing the therapeutic properties of scent. "Aroma affects your psyche. Stress symptoms like sweating, increased heart rate, and stomach cramps are controlled by hormones. Certain scents tell the brain not to release those stress hormones. A specific pleasurable scent can create a new emotional reaction to things," says aromatherapist and founder of the New York Institute of Aromatherapy Amy Galper.

Practicing aromatherapy at home is easy. Decide what you are aiming for—help with sleep or stress, for example—and choose three to five essential oils from each mood group on the opposite page. "Aroma-therapy works best when oils are combined," says Galper. To create a custom blend, combine two drops of each of your chosen three to five essential oils (10 drops maximum if you are using five essential oils) into two tablespoons (or one ounce) of olive oil (or another natural oil). You can either massage the blend into your skin or put it in a bath. As essen-tial oils are highly potent, pure chemical compounds, it's important to dilute them with olive oil before applying them to your body or adding them to a bath. You can apply your custom blend anywhere on your body, but placing it on your wrists, chest, shoulders, or neck so you can easily breathe in the scent will ensure you get the full effects. You can also try using a diffuser. A nebulizing diffuser that vaporizes the oils into a fine mist without using heat or water is best.

STRESS-BUSTERS

Floral essential oils such as lavender, rose, jasmine, ylang-ylang, and neroli calm and soothe the central nervous system, lowering the body's stress response. Flower oils contain ingredients that help you slow down and calm down emotionally.

ENERGIZERS

When you want to recharge, reach for fennel seed, rosemary, peppermint, and eucalyptus to make you feel more alert and focused. These oils also help with clearing mucus and detoxifying your system.

MOOD ELEVATORS

To help banish the blues, choose scents that are uplifting and energizing, such as citrus oils including lime, lemon, grapefruit, and sweet orange. "These oils are cleansing and detoxifying, so the physical action affects the emotional. They help body and mind let go of the negative and embrace the positive," says Galper.

SLEEP ENHANCERS

If you have any trouble relaxing and falling asleep at the end of the day, turn to lavender, clary sage, ylang-ylang, and red mandarin. Lavender has sedative qualities, clary sage and ylang-ylang relax muscles, and red mandarin works to quell nerves.

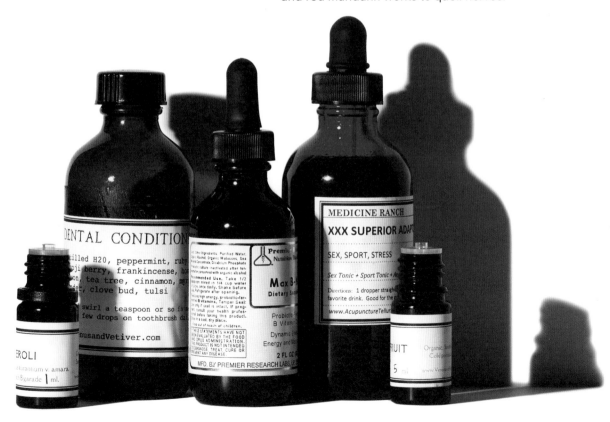

beauty sleep

When you are tired, it shows: dark circles under the eyes, dull skin, breakouts, and a loss of focus and energy. But what is enough sleep, exactly? The National Sleep Foundation recommends seven to nine hours a night for people ages 18 to 64, and about an hour less for people ages 65 and up. Functional medicine expert Dr. Ken Davis has another take. He says it's not about the number of hours, it's about how much REM cycle sleep you're getting. "If you go through four to five REM cycles, you will wake up feeling refreshed and renewed," he says. Since you can't count your REM cycles, the goal with sleep is to wake up feeling revitalized. The aim is to move through the non-REM stage (including a period of deep sleep, when your body restores tissue and muscle and strengthens bones and the immune system) into the rapid-eye-movement phase (when your brain is more active and perhaps dreaming).

Since cortisol levels should be at their highest in the morning, Davis says that's when you should have the most energy if you're sleeping well. If you can't get out of bed in the morning and have a lot of energy at 1 a.m., that means your cortisol levels are off and your sleep is not restoring your body the way it should. Consult with your doctor to check your cortisol and adrenal levels. Your doctor should be able to prescribe specific supplements and nutrients such as melatonin, magnesium, inositol, and rubidium to help get you on track. "Rubidium helps put the brakes on that overdrive in the adrenal function, and inositol is good to take before bed to calm the brain and nerves," says Davis.

Breaking your tech and TV addiction, especially before bed, is essential if you want better sleep quality. With phones constantly pinging (which immediately causes stress), it's hard to ever feel relaxed. Davis recommends unplugging two hours before bedtime. "These devices have a low-frequency electromagnetic radiation that can affect neurotransmitters and can contribute to overstimulation and anxiety," he says.

Diet and exercise affect sleep as well. Regular exercise is key, even if it is just walking. "Even walking three miles four times a week can make a difference," Davis explains. Lay off the caffeine after 2 p.m., and for alcohol, wait at least an hour after your last drink before you sleep. "Alcohol may help you fall asleep, but all the sugar in the alcohol will cause a rapid rise and then decline in your blood sugar, which will cause you to wake up."

To fall asleep more easily, develop a nighttime ritual. If possible, set a regular sleep schedule, both for when you go to bed and when you wake up. Don't take daytime naps, as it will interfere with your sleep at night. Use your bedroom only for sleep—no tech or TV. Practice deep breathing or listen to a guided relaxation app or CD. When you're getting your sleep balance right, you will feel more alert and energetic and look fresher and brighter.

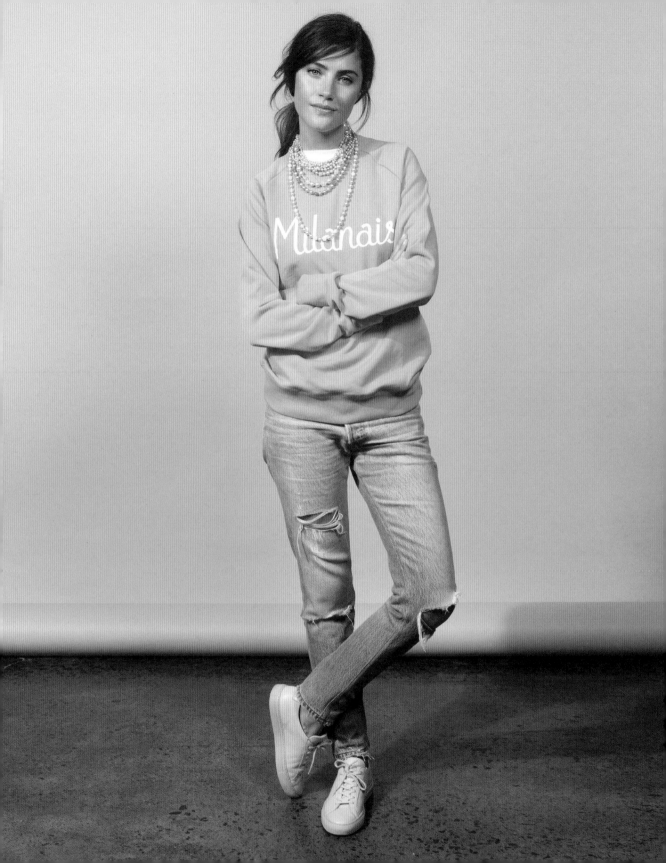

Confidence

We are all a work in progress. While some people are born confident, for most of us it takes some work. As a kid, I spent too much time wanting to look like other people, whether they were the cheerleaders, gymnasts, or just the cool girls who all happened to be tall, skinny, blonde, and blue-eyed—which I definitely was not. When I saw the movie *Love Story*, it was the first time I saw a beautiful actress who looked like me. With her dark hair, strong brows, and naturally pretty face, Ali MacGraw became my role model.

Years later, I moved to New York City and began working in the fashion industry. I was surrounded by tons of uber-tall, skinny models from all over the globe. On top of that, the stylists and fashion editors were cool and chic, hailing from Paris or London. Here I was—a kid from the Midwest and way out of my element. But I wanted in, so I became a sponge. I observed how they dressed, how they acted, and what they knew.

It took a while—until my mid-30s—to really get that I just needed to be me. I had learned to love myself exactly as I was: five feet tall, not a model, but a makeup artist who was also a suburban mom. I had a life, family, and priorities to focus on instead of fixating on what I was not. I actually remember having a big aha moment at the Met Ball, among all the celebrities, supermodels, and bold-faced names and fabulous faces. I realized I had a choice. I could feel insecure and uncomfortable or I could have a great time. I chose to dance, have fun, and just be me.

I still spend a lot of time with gorgeous women, models, actresses, and influencers from all over. I get photographed with them all, and even in my five-inch YSL Tribute heels, I'm still smaller than most. (If I'm not being photographed, I am most likely in my sneakers. I choose comfort over height nearly every time.) I take pride in my collection of photos with super-tall people—and secretly cherish my photo with Dr. Ruth, who is one of the few people I tower over.

There is a difference in people who are confident. Not only does confidence make you more attractive, it makes you feel unstoppable. There are many ways to find confidence. One of the keys is surrounding yourself with people who build you up and are there when you need them. In retrospect, many people I met in my early career became role models for how to be myself—people who thrived on being unique, such as Bruce Weber, Yogi Berra, Susan Sarandon, and Ricky Lauren. Observing them, I began to feel comfortable in my own skin. Being healthy, vibrant, and strong is another way to feel great. Above all, my secret to confidence—which is also the motto of the brand I founded—is to be who you are.

BE WHO YOU ARE

I've met so many women from all over the world, and the truth is we are all basically the same. We want to feel good, look good, and be respected, safe, and loved. Women often share with me not just their beauty issues, but also their insecurities and frustrations. While we all have these, it feels cathartic to talk about them. The secret is to move on. When you stop fighting yourself, you can then let go. The most confident—and attractive—women I know are the ones who are comfortable in their own skin. They make no apologies for who they are. They own it.

FOCUS ON WHAT'S RIGHT, NOT WHAT'S WRONG

As a makeup artist, one of the things I see all the time is that people point out their flaws before I do their face. They have a wrinkle here, an imperfection there. Usually I don't see anything. I'm focused on what makes them beautiful.

It's human nature to focus on what's not working, but usually you see imperfections about yourself that no one else sees. Truly, no one notices! Who cares if your tummy is big or you have a little pimple? No one. Everyone is too busy with their own life (and probably focused on their own flaws).

We all have something we don't like about our physical appearance. The key is to switch your focus to what is working. Play that up. It takes practice. When I look in the mirror and I notice something I'm not wild about, I try to counter it by focusing on something I do like. Besides, you have much more important things to focus on than the negative.

confidence
and social media

As a visual person I love Instagram for checking out cool destinations, beauty, food, and artists and for expressing my creative side. However, there's another dimension to social media that's not so positive: the filters and retouching that set up unattainable ideas of beauty, the obsession with selfies, and the way the whole thing encourages the comparison game and affects people's self-esteem.

Know that a lot of what you see on social media isn't real. Many social media stars have both professional photographers and retouchers on their staffs. That cute bikini photo that looks so spontaneous and perfect was probably taken at the most flattering angle possible, with some digital altering too. If you find yourself feeling bad while looking at someone's account, just stop following them. Or at least remind yourself that what you're looking at is more art than reality. Trying to get the same body, look, or life as someone else, especially when it's not real to begin with, won't ever work.

There are a lot of inspirational women out there, including Mindy Kaling, Lena Dunham, Ashley Graham, and Amy Schumer, who are rebelling against posting "perfect" pictures. They're speaking out about the damaging effects of looking at manufactured images and how it's much better to just rock individuality and see your "imperfections" as assets. Working with so many women over the years I have seen that the most beautiful people are the ones who have that magical mix of happiness, confidence, warmth, and a sense of humor. Celebrating those qualities, rather than trying to match some unattainable ideal, is a much better route.

seven cool, confident, and inspiring women

———

Through my work, I've met so many incredible women—from trailblazers to CEOs, writers, designers, moms, doctors, athletes, and teachers (to name a few). I'm always inspired by women who do what they love, sometimes overcoming hurdles and breaking barriers to get where they are. I try to learn from them about what they do to feel great. From Gabby Reece to Laila Ali, here are the stories of seven inspiring, successful women and their thoughts on confidence, challenges, health, and beauty.

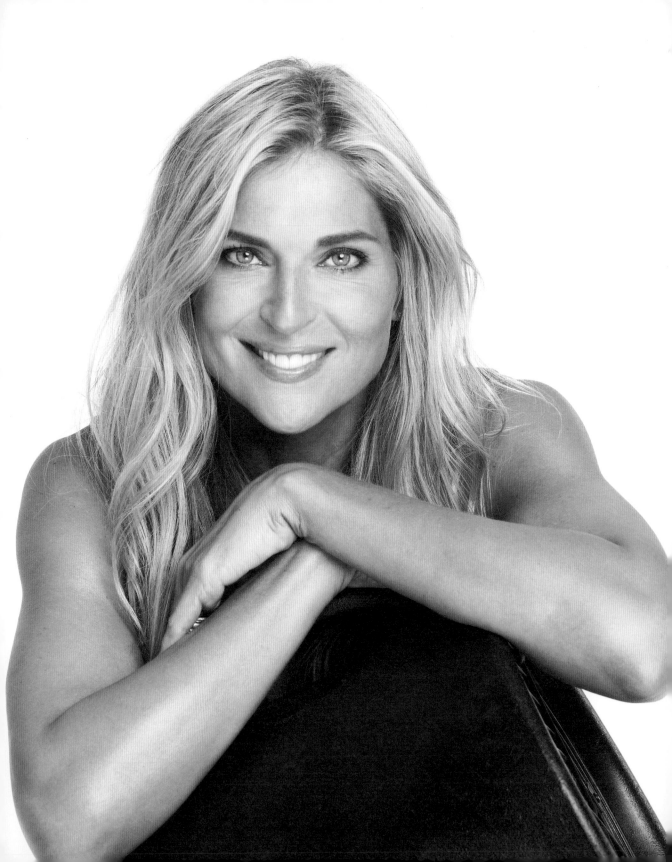

Gabby Reece

Before Gabby Reece became a fitness guru, before she was one of the world's best pro volleyball players, before she married Laird Hamilton and became a mom of three girls, she started out as a model. We met on photo shoots in the late '80s, when I did her makeup for British and Italian *Vogue*. I loved how funny, honest, and totally real she is. We could not have been more opposite in appearance—she is blonde and 6'3"—but we shared a passion for health and fitness. Reece has turned that passion into her career and is an inspiring example of how strong is beautiful.

WHAT IS YOUR BEST BEAUTY TIP?

My number-one beauty tip is happiness. Your skin is an outer reflection of your overall inner well-being. I have three daughters, so stress is unavoidable. Whether you're working or you have a family, these are things you care about and they create stress. I try to ask myself, "Is this really worth getting worked up about?" If it's not, then I back away from the emotion quickly. I believe there is a way in relationships to healthily express your feelings right away and not hold things in too much. The exercise and the healthy eating I practice don't only make me feel good, they're also a positive way of handling stress.

WHAT ARE YOUR GO-TO WORKOUTS RIGHT NOW?

I do high-intensity circuit training three days a week. In the summer, three days a week, I do ballistic pool training underwater with weights, which is a way to work really hard without beating up your body. It's another form of strength training that's easier on your muscles, bones, and tendons. As you get older, the more you can do high-intensity training—short bursts of high-energy workouts—or ballistic training, the better.

WHAT ARE YOUR BEAUTY-FROM-THE-INSIDE TIPS?

Omega supplements are very good for your skin. I take them daily. Blue-green algae is also good for skin. It doesn't taste the best (it tastes like seaweed), but if you can just do a shot of it a few times a week, you'll see results.

HOW DO YOU FIND CONFIDENCE ON THOSE DAYS WHEN YOU JUST DON'T FEEL IT?

You can influence how you're feeling by adjusting your physical posture. On the days I actually don't feel my best, I will go out of my way to overexaggerate standing upright and walking in a commanding way, because this can shift how you are feeling. If you're feeling low and you hunch over and you close your shoulders, you are creating a physiological response in your body. We can help ourselves with a few little changes in our posture; there is a lot of science to support that.

YOU LIVE IN HAWAII AND ARE OUT IN THE SUN OFTEN. HOW DO YOU PROTECT YOUR SKIN?

I'm not a big sun worshipper even though I'm outside a lot. But a little bit of sun every day is not bad for us. I think it's important to moderate, protecting yourself from the sun while also being in the sun to get vitamin D. Once or twice a year, I get micro-dermabrasion to kind of sandblast off some of the dead skin. I'm of the school of less is more.

WHAT IS THE BIGGEST CHALLENGE YOU'VE FACED AND HOW DID YOU OVERCOME IT?

When I was a young kid, I ended up living with friends of my mother's for about five years, and in that time, my father passed away. Until I was about 17, my life wasn't the easiest. But I always say that we are dealt high cards and low cards and there comes a point where if you can appreciate what the low cards have taught you and also have gratitude and awareness of your high cards, that's a hand to be happy with. It's just about maintaining perspective—to really stay focused on what is good, or what gifts you have been given. You can always find something.

"My number-one beauty tip is happiness."

Hannah Bronfman

Hannah is one of those people who seems to have nonstop energy. She's warm, open, and always smiling. Hannah co-founded the Beautified app, which helps people book last-minute beauty appointments. She's also an in-demand DJ around the globe. It's no surprise that she's built up a huge following on Instagram and her lifestyle site, HBFIT .com, where she focuses on fitness, healthy living, and beauty.

WHEN DID FITNESS BECOME A PART OF YOUR LIFE?

I was a dancer until I was 16, and then I played team sports in high school and I kept very active in college. When my grandmother passed away—she suffered from anorexia her whole life—it was just one of those experiences that led me to devote myself to living a happy and healthy lifestyle, one that she was never able to live for herself. That loss is what started me on my journey of self-exploration and self-love when I was in college.

WHY IS MIXING UP YOUR WORKOUTS SO IMPORTANT FOR YOU?

Keeping a balance between different workouts is the key for me. If I'm working out five times a week, I love to do some-thing different every day. Whether that's Pilates or boxing or taking a dance class or trampoline class or lifting weights with my trainer, I really like to switch it up all the time so I don't get bored. My feeling is that if my body is never getting used to one thing, it's constantly working.

"WORK HARD, PLAY HARD" IS ONE OF YOUR MOTTOS; WHAT DOES THAT MEAN FOR YOU?

It's a term that I live my life by. I work really hard, whether it's in the gym or in my job—I definitely put a lot of energy and focus into those aspects of my life. But I also love to entertain and be out with friends. I'm a really social person and I love being around people. I think it's important to enjoy the downtime that I have, and take advantage of every moment.

WHAT ARE YOUR FAVORITE BEAUTY FOODS?

Matcha is one of them. The powder form of green tea gives me sustained energy levels without any crashing, and it's full of antioxidants and vitamin A, so it's very clarifying. I also put two tablespoons of Great Lakes Gelatin collagen in my hot or cold smoothies. The elasticity in my skin has definitely changed over time just by ingesting collagen. I would say that chlorophyll is another one. You can get chlorophyll in liquid form or liquid gel capsule form—I like the liquid form. I put two droppers in a liter and a half of water and drink it. It's really good for your blood, for your skin, for your digestive system. The other beauty booster is water. When I consume three liters of water a day, I completely notice that my undereyes don't look as tired, even if I haven't had enough sleep.

YOU'RE VERY HEALTH-CONSCIOUS, BUT WHAT ARE YOUR CHEATS? COCKTAILS? SWEETS?

I'm a big fan of living a guilt-free life. I think we all work really hard during the day on our bodies and on our minds, and if having a drink at night is part of your lifestyle, that's okay. I don't think that that's something to be ashamed of or to be frowned upon. I'm a tequila drinker and I usually drink it without anything in it. Just some lime and ice because I don't want to drink a lot of sugar at night. I also love a margarita and I love rosé in the summer. I try not to feel guilty if I'm munching on something late at night or have pizza once in a while. Everything in moderation.

"loss is what started me on my journey of self-exploration and self-love."

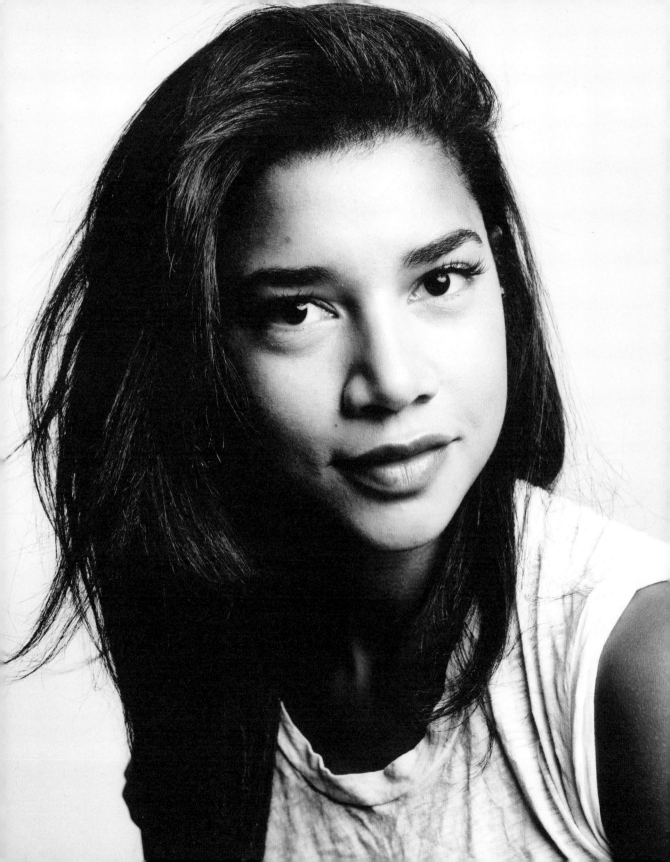

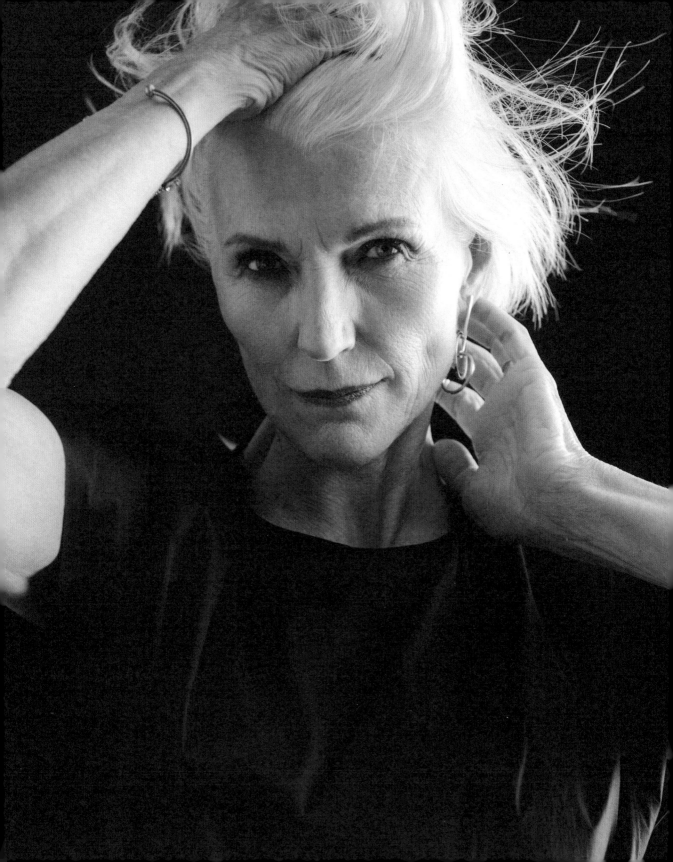

Maye Musk

At 68, model Maye Musk is busier than ever. Having modeled since she was 15, Maye decided to let her gray grow out at 60 and has had some of her biggest career success recently: booking the covers of *Elle Québec*, *Time*, and *New York Magazine*. But modeling isn't Maye's only job; she is also a successful nutritionist and living proof of the strong link between health and beauty. Maye has balanced both careers as a single mother raising her three children: filmmaker Tosca Musk, entrepreneur Kimbal Musk, and Tesla CEO Elon Musk.

WHEN DID YOU FIRST REALIZE THAT NUTRITION AND BEAUTY OVERLAPPED?

Originally, I never thought they overlapped. I kept my nutrition business and modeling separate. Now that I'm over 60, they are overlapping more than ever. It's important to have good health and plenty of energy for modeling and speaking engagements. On photo shoots, younger models love chatting with me. The biggest difficulty is maintaining weight. We need to eat well most of the time. Temptation is everywhere!

WHAT ARE YOUR FAVORITE BEAUTY FOODS?

Foods that people are terrified to eat due to myths and fad diets: fruits and vegetables, milk and yogurt, whole wheat bread, cereal and potatoes, legumes and nuts.

DO YOU EVER CHEAT?

Yes, I have a sweet tooth! Chocolates and sweet foods are tempting and require a good deal of restraint in order for me to avoid overindulging. When my friends order dessert, I warn them that I'll probably eat most of their dishes. After that, I eat perfectly for the next few days.

WHAT DO YOU DO FOR OVERALL WELLNESS?

I plan my meals and snacks in order to prevent hunger. If you get hungry, you'll eat anything! I always have nutritious foods at home and try to order carefully when out. It's not easy, but it's essential. As you get older, overeating punishes you more and for longer.

WHAT DO YOU DO TO STAY FIT AND STRONG?

I walk my dog four times a day. About five times a week I'll do the treadmill, stationary bike, or swim for 30 minutes. I use weights every other day and also do stretches. I don't push myself hard because it can cause me pain. When modeling in large cities, I like to walk to the job—sightseeing while exercising.

YOU'VE BEEN A MODEL FOR OVER FIVE DECADES. WHAT DO YOU THINK HAS BEEN THE KEY TO YOUR LONGEVITY?

Maintaining weight is important. Now I'm a size 6. During the '80s I was a plus-size model. I was tired of watching my diet and thought about giving up modeling, which didn't end up happening, as plus-size modeling was in demand at that time. There is a lot of rejection in modeling; that's part of the industry. You just have to be able to cope and move on. I had a busy nutrition practice and traveled the world as a wellness speaker, so the rejection didn't bother me.

WHAT IS THE BEST BEAUTY TIP YOU HAVE FOR WOMEN IN THEIR 60S?

Stay out of the sun or cover yourself up.

WHAT IS THE BEST BEAUTY TIP YOU'VE LEARNED OVERALL?

Be happy, stay positive, and smile.

WHEN AND HOW DID YOU FIND YOUR CONFIDENCE?

My siblings and I grew up confident because we had wonderful parents. This confidence got knocked out of me many times. I just kept going to survive. Everyone has had tragedies, but thinking about them and dwelling on them makes you miserable. I have my confidence back now. The 60s are great.

"It's important to have good health and plenty of energy."

Cassandra Grey

Cassandra Grey has merged tech, Hollywood, and the beauty industry with her site Violet Grey. It was a smart move that's turned into one of the coolest online destinations. Along with a chic virtual magazine called *The Violet Files*, the site features an edited collection of the best products chosen by beauty insiders and Hollywood makeup artists. Everything feels modern, glamorous, and perfectly curated, just like Cassandra's own style.

WHEN IT COMES TO MAKEUP, WHAT'S THE BEST TRICK YOU'VE LEARNED OVER THE YEARS?

Brush your teeth with French baking soda to whiten your teeth. Clean and pretty teeth are everything.

WHAT BEAUTY TREATMENTS HAVE YOU DONE THAT REALLY MAKE A DIFFERENCE? WHY DO YOU LOVE THEM?

Nano-current facials really make a difference. Sunday-night massages are great for your skin.

WHAT HAVE YOU LEARNED ABOUT BEAUTY FROM BEING IN THE BEAUTY BUSINESS?

It is the self-esteem business.

WHAT ARE YOUR FAVORITE BEAUTY FOODS?

Avocado, coconut oil, and lemon water.

WHAT DO YOU LOVE THAT'S NOT HEALTHY?

Flying across the pond, grilled cheese, and pancakes.

WHAT DO YOU DO FOR WELLNESS?

Read a lot. Sleep a lot.

WHAT DO YOU DO TO STAY STRONG?

Love my family.

WHAT DO YOU DO TO FEEL CONFIDENT ON THOSE DAYS YOU DON'T?

Let my family love me.

WHAT'S THE BIGGEST HURDLE YOU'VE
OVERCOME IN YOUR LIFE AND HOW
DID YOU DO IT?

I started at the bottom. Hard work is the
secret sauce, ladies and gentlemen. The
opening line in *The Departed* is something
like this, which pretty much sums up my
aspirations: "I don't want to be a product of
my environment, I want my environment to
be a product of me."

*"Hard work is the
secret sauce."*

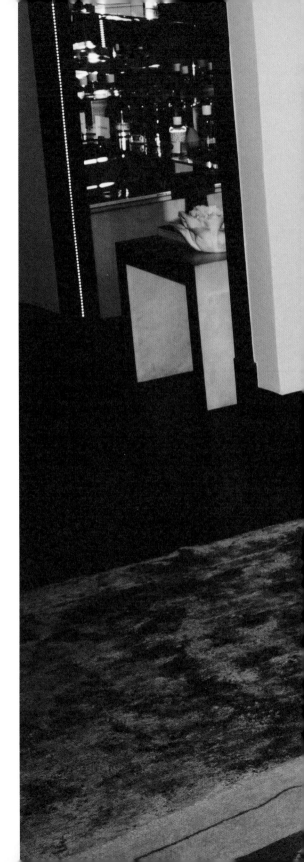

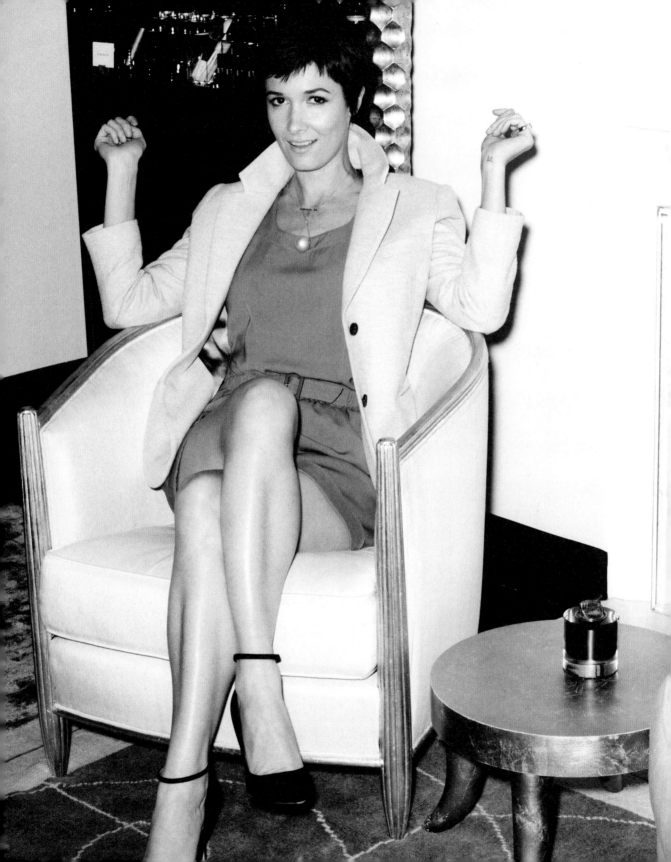

Elle Macpherson

If you check out Elle Macpherson's Instagram account, you can see why she was nicknamed "The Body." Now in her 50s, she looks as incredible as ever. I've known her since the '90s, and the former supermodel-turned-entrepreneur has always been into fitness and health. Elle credits her age-defying looks to eating alkaline. She started the diet when she met Dr. Simone Laubscher, whom she's partnered with to create a health and wellness product company called WelleCo. The busy mom of two has started a business that reflects her belief that beauty comes from within, explaining: "I know if I nourish my cells from the inside, it will show on the outside."

YOU ARE ON AN ALKALINE DIET. HOW IS THAT DIFFERENT THAN JUST EATING HEALTHIER?

Eating alkaline means eating more plants and fewer animals, which sounds easy but can actually be tricky. Due to my busy schedule and frequent traveling through different time zones, sometimes I struggle to find a healthy food option. I take the WelleCo Alkalising Greens supplement because it's a simple and effective option and is vegan, organic, and gluten free. The supplement helps to keep me strong and well-nourished with vitamins, minerals, and probiotics all in one.

WHAT IS THE CONNECTION BETWEEN THE ALKALINE DIET AND BEAUTY?

The alkalinity of your body informs your pH level, the balance of which is essential to overall well-being. I've been told the ideal alkaline range is 6.5 to 7.5. However, modern lifestyle and a diet heavy in dairy, red meat, and processed foods can upset the body's healthy pH balance. Many of us are off-balance and too acidic, which causes health issues big and small. After taking the Alkalising Greens every day I began to notice that my skin wasn't dry anymore, looked plumper, and had what nutritionists call "the alkaline glow." The skin is a great barometer of how you are feeling inside.

WHAT ARE YOUR FAVORITE BEAUTY FOODS?

Water first and foremost! I love green vegetables and beets and avocado. Also most types of fruit, including mango, papaya, blackberries, and coconuts, which are all full of antioxidants and vitamins, low in fats and calories, and a delicious sweet treat on a summer's day.

I KNOW YOU HAVE EXPLORED A LOT OF ALTERNATIVE THERAPIES. WHICH ONES HAVE HAD THE MOST IMPACT?

Aromatherapy is wonderful for calming nerves and creating a sense of peace.

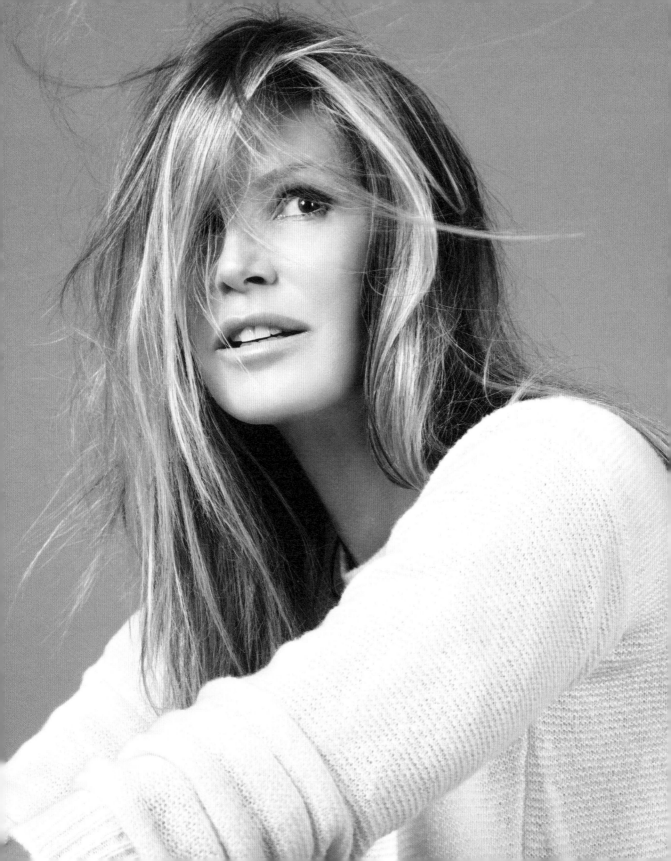

WHAT DO YOU DO TO STAY STRONG?

I define myself by my joy factor, so I do physical activities that make my heart sing. In my spare time I love skiing, swimming, or hiking; just getting outdoors and enjoying nature.

WHAT DO YOU DO TO FEEL CONFIDENT ON THOSE DAYS WHEN YOU DON'T FEEL IT?

I dedicate about 30 minutes every morning to meditation. I find it helps keep me balanced so I feel strong and confident. At the end of the day I make sure I get a good night's sleep to energize myself for the next day. Happiness and wellness is my ultimate goal.

WHAT'S THE BIGGEST HURDLE YOU'VE OVERCOME IN YOUR LIFE AND HOW DID YOU DO IT?

To believe in myself. At 52, I now know that confidence comes from wisdom, intuition, experience, and love.

WHEN IT COMES TO MAKEUP, WHAT'S THE BEST TRICK YOU'VE LEARNED OVER THE YEARS?

Less is more. If you are healthy, your skin is healthy, you need less makeup, and you will radiate with a natural glow. I also choose makeup products that are sheer. That's why I love the Bobbi Brown lip glosses—they are light and natural. I also use brow pencil. As a blonde, filling in my brows with the pencil brings a bit of definition to frame my eyes.

"At 52, I now know that confidence comes from wisdom, intuition, experience, and love."

Olivia Munn

When I first interviewed Olivia Munn, we clicked. She was driving in LA and I was in my bedroom in New Jersey and we chatted about everything. I love how candid, open, and funny Olivia is. She's also super-inspiring. She has a black belt in tae kwon do, an amazing boyfriend who happens to be the quarterback for the Green Bay Packers, and a successful acting and producing career, and she is as down-to-earth as they come. She's in kickass shape thanks to mastering incredible fitness challenges for her movies. Olivia is always researching the next big thing in beauty, including eating foods that contain hyaluronic acid. Talk about beauty from the inside out!

WHAT MOVES OR WORKOUTS DID YOU LEARN ON SETS THAT YOU LOVE?

I got into great shape on *X-Men* without thinking about what I looked like physically. My goals every day were to learn a new skill or move. The side effect was the weight loss and the muscle tone. My brain was doing the workout, but my body was getting the results. And I think that's the kind of workout that works best for me. I don't want to think about what I look like or about fitting into a certain pair of jeans. Instead, I like to think about getting as fit, healthy, and strong as I possibly can, because if that's your goal, everything else falls into place.

IS IT TRUE THAT A HYPNOTIST GOT YOU TO LOVE WORKING OUT?

That's true. I was always very active growing up doing gymnastics, cheerleading, and tae kwon do. Training for those kinds of sports was more goal-based. If I wanted to do a spinning back kick, I would just break down the move and learn to do it. So

basically I never created the pathways in my brain to motivate and go for a run or lift weights. Seeing the hypnotist helped motivate me to start working out, because I had no motivation. Even the thought of looking leaner or more toned wasn't enough for me to work out, but I knew that I wanted to be fit. Wanting something and finding the motivation to do it can be very separate for me at times.

HOW DO FITNESS AND BEAUTY OVERLAP FOR YOU?

Before *X-Men*, I wouldn't overlap them. But now I can't separate them. Being in shape makes me feel powerful because I know that no matter what life may throw at me, I have given myself the best chance to conquer it—not just physically, but mentally, too. When I've learned to jump or kick or balance, I've gained the confidence and practice to face any obstacle. And on the beauty side of it, when you work out, new blood flow circulates through your body and your face. Studies show that

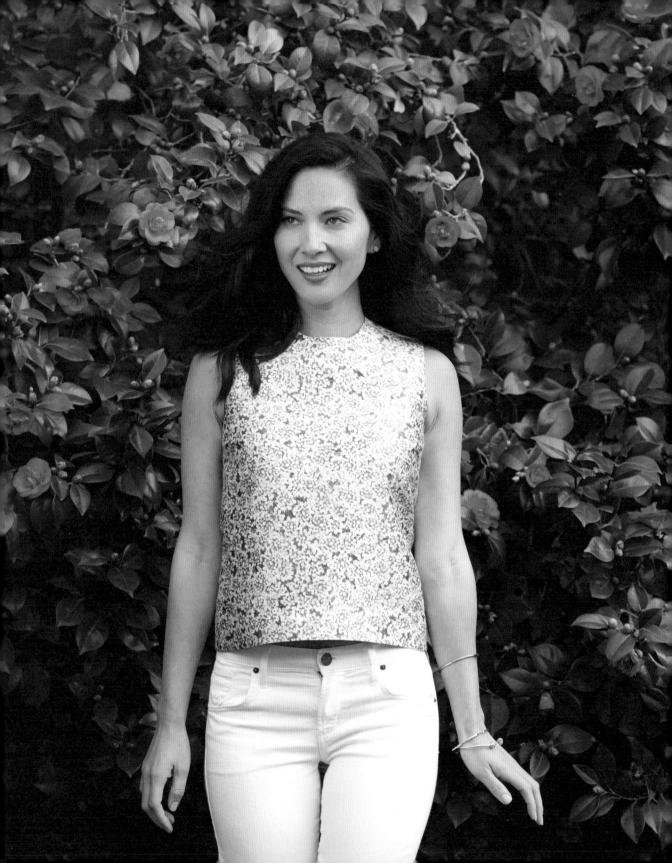

new blood circulation helps to slow the aging process, which gives your skin more elasticity and suppleness.

WHAT BEAUTY TREATMENTS HAVE YOU TRIED? WHAT REALLY WORKS AND WHAT DOESN'T?

I've done Ultherapy, which is a laser treatment that's supposed to go deep into your skin and help reproduce collagen. You can see the results best on people whose skin has already dropped, so I'm not sure if it really worked on me. I've only done it once and it hurt so badly. On a scale of 1 to 10, it was a 15. It felt like someone was taking a hot iron to my face and holding it for five seconds over and over and over. They said I should do it once a year to keep aging away, but I'm not sure I could go through that pain again.

WHAT ARE YOUR FAVORITE BEAUTY FOODS?

I'm a big believer in the foods we eat being able to reverse the clock or speed it up. I love eating anything with hyaluronic acid in it: okra, mangos, cilantro, certain potatoes. Removing sunspots is a big anti-ager. I have freckles and I love them, but there's a difference between a sunspot and a freckle. I use dark-mark fading pads every night to help diminish the extra sun I got during the day and help keep my skin tone even.

"Being in shape makes me feel powerful because I know that no matter what life may throw at me, I have given myself the best chance to conquer it—not just physically, but mentally, too. When I've learned to jump or kick or balance, I've gained the confidence and practice to face any obstacle."

WHAT'S THE BIGGEST HURDLE YOU'VE OVERCOME IN YOUR LIFE AND HOW DID YOU DO IT?

My anxiety is something that I'm continuing to overcome. I've made great strides in the last year or so, and I'm very proud of myself for that. My anxiety manifests itself in OCD and trichotillomania. People who live with anxiety understand when I say that it's a tiring journey. To commit to changing is not as easy as it sounds. But I'm figuring out ways to do it, sometimes just inches at a time. By not forcing myself to change overnight and allowing myself to go a little bit at a time or even stand still in my progress, I've been able to hold on to my progress. That's been my greatest achievement, I think—the tiny steps I've made to slowly rid my life of anxiety.

WHAT'S THE BEST MAKEUP TRICK YOU'VE LEARNED ON A MOVIE SET?

Putting my concealer under my eyes in an upside-down triangle before foundation. It helps draw the light to your eyes.

WHAT IS YOUR MAKEUP GO-TO WHEN YOU'RE HAVING A BAD BEAUTY DAY?

I call it "doll face." When I want to feel pretty, I do a full face with blush, eyebrows, and a pretty stained lip. When the lips and the blush are almost identical, it makes your face look really fresh and pulled together, like a little doll face.

Laila Ali

There's something amazing about a woman who can hold her own in a boxing ring. Being a four-time world champion without even playing sports as a child—that's even more incredible. That's Laila Ali. The daughter of boxing legend Muhammad Ali, Laila took her own successful turn in the ring and is now a wellness and fitness expert. Smart, gorgeous, poised, and very cool, Laila is an example of how health, beauty, and confidence are intertwined.

WHAT DID YOU LEARN ABOUT YOURSELF DURING YOUR BOXING CAREER? HOW DID IT SHAPE YOUR PERCEPTION OF YOURSELF?

I learned that I am an athlete. I never participated in sports growing up, so boxing taught me that by being disciplined, focused, and dedicated, I can do anything I desire. Because of boxing, I will always see myself as a champion . . . physically and mentally.

HAVE YOU ALWAYS BEEN CONFIDENT?

I have always been more confident than the average person. I think growing up in a household with parents that didn't put limits on me helped me develop a confident mind and a positive perception of myself. I realized at an early age that everyone makes mistakes and there is no such thing as "perfect." This realization freed me from being afraid to express myself due to fear of failure.

WHAT ARE YOUR GO-TO WORKOUTS NOW THAT YOU AREN'T IN THE RING?

I like to mix it up! When I work out I like to sweat and push myself so that I see and feel results. I run, spin, sprint, and do the StairMaster. I also hit the heavy bag, use free weights, and do abdominal workouts. I keep working until I get a good sweat and burn going. I try to do at least 60 minutes, four days a week.

WHAT ARE THE FOODS THAT FUEL YOU?

I like to do superfood protein shakes because it's the easiest way to get my daily dose of the nutrients my body needs. I mix in blueberries, spinach, coconut oil, protein, avocado, chlorella, maca powder, and cacao powder. I also love sweet potatoes for energy!

IS THERE ONE BEAUTY LOOK THAT MAKES YOU FEEL THE MOST CONFIDENT?

I feel most confident when my skin looks clear, even, and hydrated.

WHAT IS YOUR BEAUTY ROUTINE WHEN YOU HAVE ONLY FIVE MINUTES?

My beauty routine is simple. It begins with a clean, moisturized face. Then I apply tinted sunscreen, mascara, and lip gloss!

WHAT'S THE BIGGEST HURDLE YOU'VE OVERCOME IN YOUR LIFE AND HOW DID YOU DO IT?

My biggest challenge in life has been slowing down mentally and physically so that I can be present, mindful, and engaged in the moment. Sometimes I am so busy multitasking and being pulled in different directions that I get anxiety and feel overwhelmed. Practicing daily meditation has made a big difference in my life and is helping me manage my busy lifestyle so I am able to execute my goals and responsibilities, while being at peace within. But this is definitely an ongoing process!

"Because of boxing, I will always see myself as a champion ... physically and mentally."

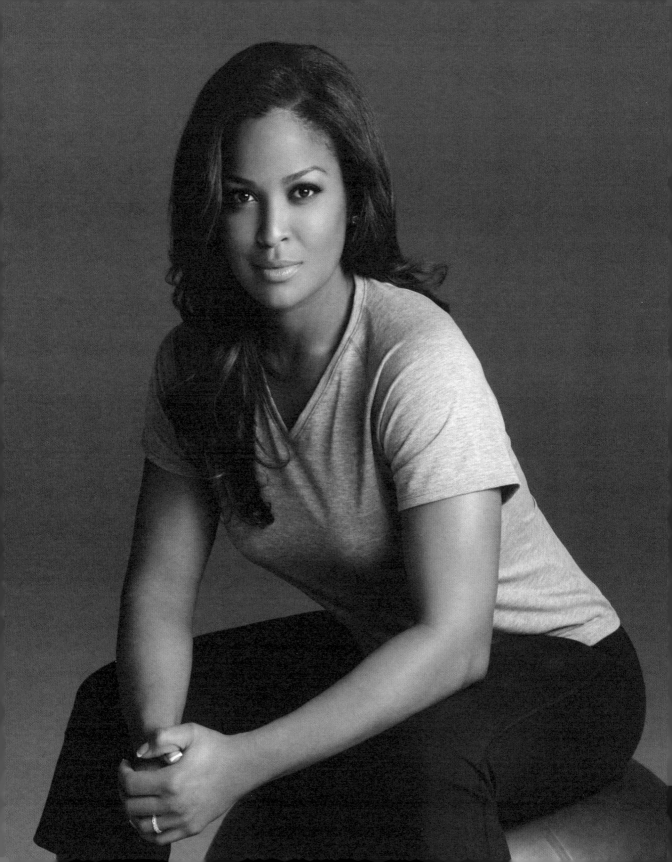

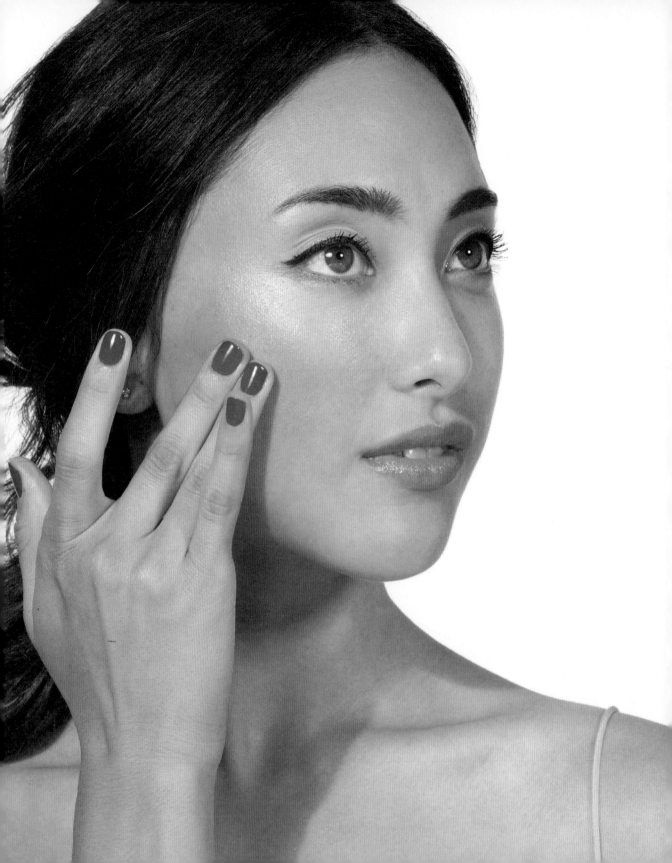

The Skin You're In

What's most beautiful to me is healthy skin. Glowing skin comes from the combination of good genes and a healthy lifestyle. I have seen firsthand how ignoring your health shows up on your face. Young, beautiful models who are bright-eyed and fresh-faced can look tired and drawn just one year later. Smoking, drugs, and too much bad food can make even a gorgeous 18-year-old look awful. I have also seen the reverse in people who decide to start eating clean and exercising and then begin to look and feel drastically better.

My advice is simple: drink enough water, get enough sleep, eat mostly beauty foods, exercise to break a sweat, and learn how to take good care of your changing skin. Layering products is an effective way to improve your skin. As health and beauty are linked, when you have a skin issue, a nutritionist can be just as helpful as a dermatologist. Here's my best advice, along with tips from a team of experts, to simplify your skincare routine, sort through the hype, use the best ingredients, and discover healthy skin.

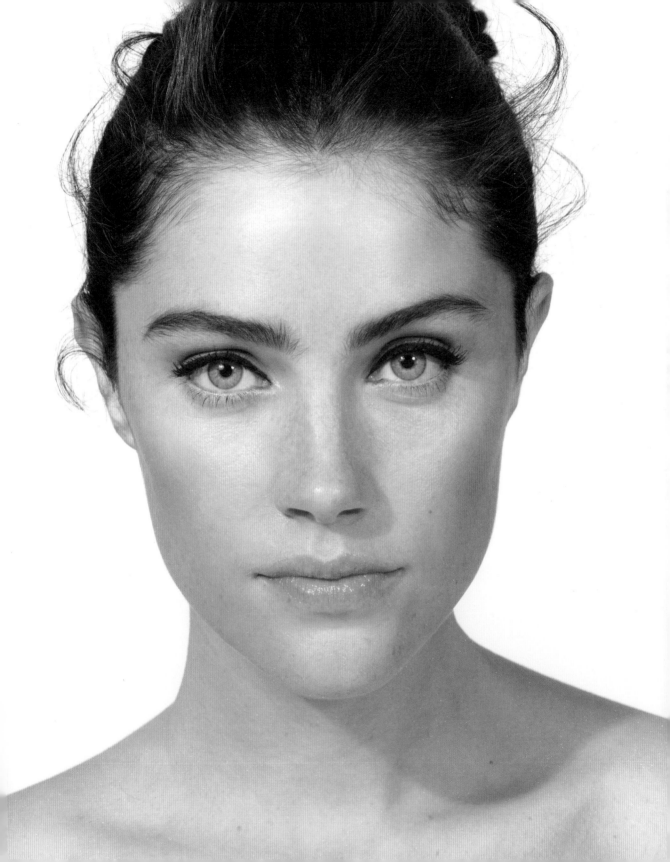

the most potent skincare ingredients

A DERMATOLOGIST WEIGHS IN

To help you navigate what really works, Manhattan-based dermatologist Dr. Sejal Shah shares eight of the most powerful skincare ingredients that can actually transform skin.

Growth factors

Peptides

Hyaluronic Acid

Hydroxy Acids

Natural Oils

Retinol

Vitamin C

Vitamin B3

GROWTH FACTORS AND PEPTIDES

Both of these ingredients have the power to repair and regenerate skin. They are found together in many anti-aging skin creams. Apply these creams twice a day to promote collagen and elastin production. Skin texture will noticeably improve after consistent use.

HYALURONIC ACID

While hyaluronic acid is the main ingredient in injectable fillers such as Juvéderm and Restylane, it can also be found in topical undereye, face, and body creams and gels. Apply a product containing hyaluronic acid to the skin and you will see an immediate change—lines soften and skin looks noticeably plumper. This is because hyaluronic acid is a normal component in your skin that helps retain moisture. The immediate plumping effect only lasts while the product is on the skin. However, softer and smoother skin is a benefit of regular use given hyaluronic acid's anti-inflammatory and skin-repairing effects.

HYDROXY ACIDS

Whether you want to soften fine lines or are battling clogged pores, alpha hydroxy acids and beta hydroxy acids are key for renewing skin. Found in serums and moisturizers, they speed cell turnover, helping skin slough off surface layers to reveal fresh, new skin underneath.

NATURAL OILS: AVOCADO, MARULA, OLIVE, GRAPESEED, AND OTHERS

These are incredibly hydrating natural oils that can restore and renew dry, sensitive skin. They have rich fatty acids that will build up your skin barrier. If you prefer chemical-free products, any of these are an excellent choice. You can apply oil directly to your skin with your fingers or a cotton swab. Use them all over your body, or just target dry patches such as heels, elbows, and cuticles.

RETINOL

A tried and true anti-aging ingredient, retinol increases collagen and elastin production, reduces hyperpigmentation, and promotes cell turnover by exfoliating skin. This is definitely a product that works better at night because it can break down when exposed to the sun. As retinol can be irritating for some, start by applying it every other night until your skin gets used to it. You need only a dime-size amount. At night, combine retinol with soothing creams that have growth factors, peptides, or vitamin B3 to hydrate and soothe skin.

Over-the-counter versions are a good place to start since they are milder than prescription-strength versions.

VITAMIN C

This antioxidant brightens skin, calms inflammation, improves the appearance of fine lines and wrinkles, reduces hyperpigmentation, and protects and repairs skin from free radical damage. It is a wonder ingredient. When layered underneath sunscreen and applied daily, the SPF will protect you from ultraviolet radiation, and the vitamin C will counteract any sun damage. Look for vitamin C concentrate or serums that come in dark bottles with a pump, so there is limited exposure to air and light (both of which can make vitamin C less effective). The more potent versions tend to be the more expensive ones and are worth splurging on.

VITAMIN B3

Vitamin B3 (a.k.a. niacinamide) is great for very sensitive skin, as it is an anti-inflammatory and anti-irritant. It can also help with general redness, discoloration, and rebuilding the skin's protective barrier so that skin looks healthier, brighter, and more hydrated overall.

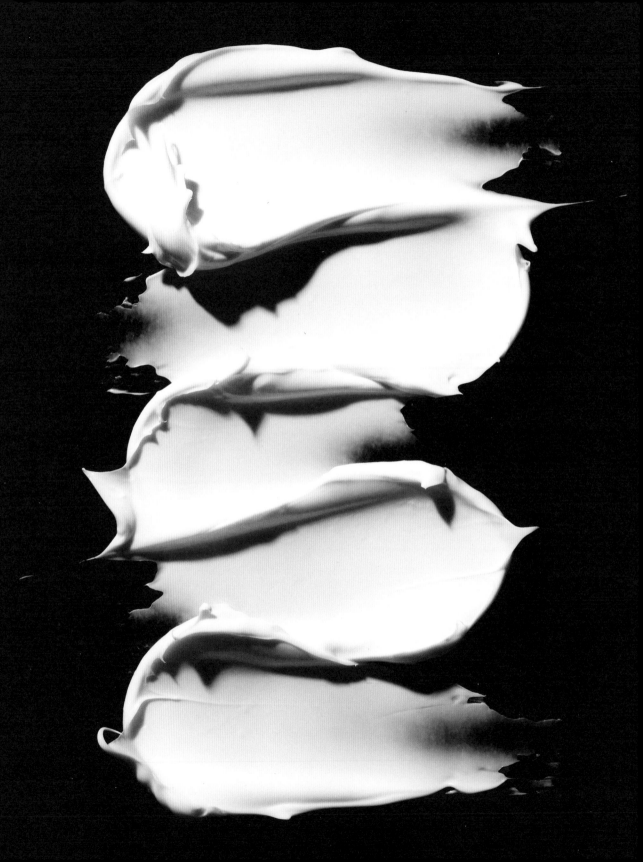

your skincare arsenal

Since your skin changes daily due to lifestyle and environment, the products you use each day should also change. Have a few different formulas on hand for when your skin needs extra help. Start with a cleanser that cleans your skin without stripping it. Even if you are oily, your skin should not feel tight after washing (a sign your cleanser is too harsh). For dry days or when your skin feels extra dehydrated, either switch up your moisturizers to creamier and more emollient ones or layer a few products to get softer skin. I love to start light with a cream that absorbs quickly and hydrates the lower layers. I sometimes add a balm on top, and I have been known to even pat a bit of oil over that as well. There are a plethora of products and formulas out there. Here is a simple breakdown of my essential products and what each does.

TONERS AND TONICS

To soothe, hydrate, or reduce oil buildup on skin, toners (sometimes called tonics) are the second step after cleansing. Avoid alcohol-based toners, which can strip and irritate the skin, even if you are oily. Look for water-based formulas with calming ingredients such as aloe, lavender, and cucumber.

SERUMS

Packed full of skin-transforming active ingredients, serums are potent weapons in your skincare routine. More potent than your average moisturizer, serums should be targeted to your skincare needs. You'll find versions for correcting acne, lifting skin, reducing fine lines, or simply creating an overall glow. Layer these on immediately after cleansing and toning and before applying any other products to make sure the active ingredients are fully absorbed into your skin. You'll notice that they immediately smooth the skin surface, but although your skin may feel hydrated, you will still need a moisturizer on top.

OILS

Don't be afraid of oils. It's a myth that oils clog your skin, or that
oils won't work with oily skin. They are wonderful for any type,
making skin look more luminous and adding a dose of intense
moisture that you can't get from creams or balms. You can use oils
on your face and body. For the body, apply it right after you get out
of the shower to towel-dried skin. For the face, layer it underneath
your moisturizing cream to deliver intense moisturizing benefits,
or just pat a small amount onto cheeks after moisturizing for an
added glow. I also use it as a refresher at the end of the day to add
moisture back to the skin after a long day wearing makeup.

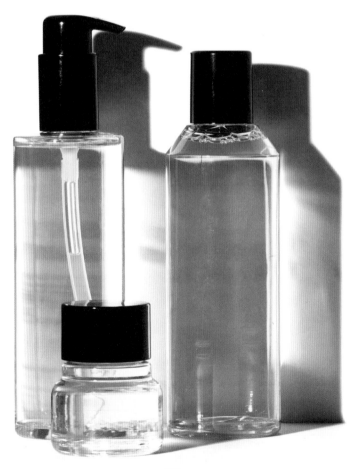

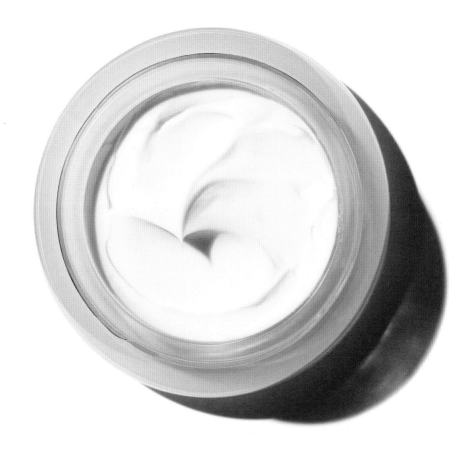

CREAMS

Every woman should have go-to day and night creams that leave skin beautifully hydrated, plump, and smooth. A good daytime moisturizer should be easily absorbed, providing a perfect canvas for makeup, and it should also deliver SPF protection. Night creams tend to be thicker and heavier and provide more intensive hydration and anti-aging ingredients.

BALMS

When you are battling ultra-dry skin, you need a balm. A rich oil-in-water emulsion boosts skin's moisture levels to create firmer, denser, smoother skin. Balms can be used as a night cream or even as a day cream during harsh winter months.

CLEANSERS

A cleanser's job is to remove dirt, makeup, and impurities. Bar soap is too drying for most people. Look instead for a milky cream, gel, balm, or oil cleanser. I love when they foam and are easy to wash off with warm water. Some will remove mascara and eye makeup, but often a separate eye makeup remover is helpful to apply before you cleanse to really get everything off. A long-wear makeup remover is a must for waterproof products.

EXFOLIANTS

No matter what type of skin you have, you need to exfoliate to reveal fresher, smoother skin. It also allows moisturizers to penetrate more effectively so your skin is soft and healthy. For your face, choose a gentle exfoliator. Exfoliating gels and masks tend to be less abrasive than scrubs on delicate facial skin. For the body, an oil paired with sea salt or brown sugar is a great go-to. I recommend exfoliating the face once or twice a week and the body as often as needed to keep your body smoothed and moisturized.

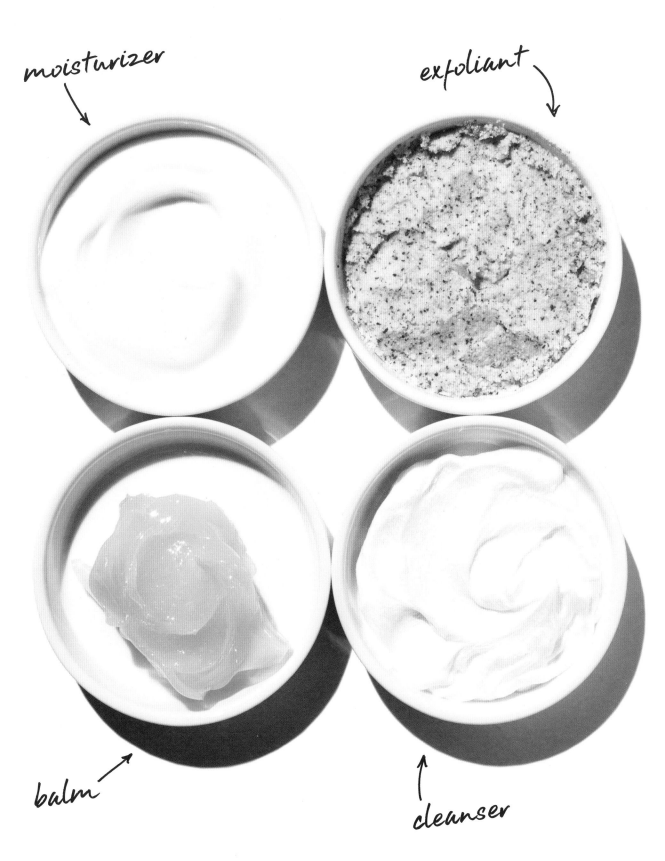

moisturizer

exfoliant

balm

cleanser

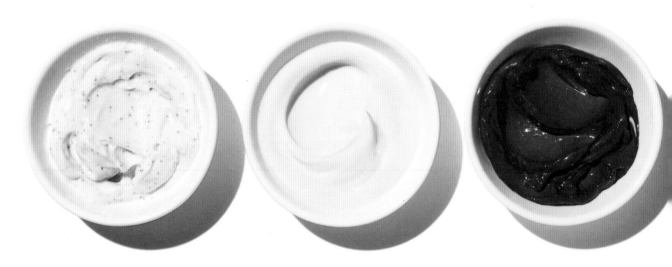

MASKS

Once a week I like to do a mini-facial at home with a great mask. Days where my pores seem clogged, I reach for a purifying clay mask that removes excess oil and pore-clogging debris. An exfoliating mask sloughs off dead skin cells to reveal beautiful smoother and tighter skin below. A hydrating mask quenches dry skin for a softer, more even finish.

REMEDIES

While food, herbs, and vitamins deliver beauty from the inside out, those ingredients can also be potent when applied topically. This is why I launched Remedies, a collection of natural-ingredient super-blends that target specific skin concerns. A few drops of each tincture applied after cleansing targets a variety of underlying issues. For example, parched skin benefits from a hyaluronic acid complex. Irritated skin is calmed with red algae. Acne-clogged skin can gain clarity and oil control thanks to a formula with manuka oil, sea buckthorn, saw palmetto, rosehip oils, and salicylic acid.

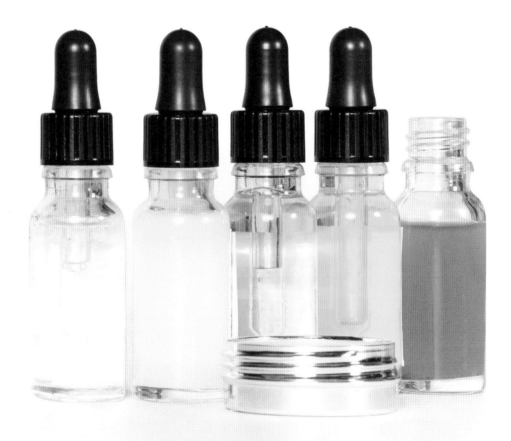

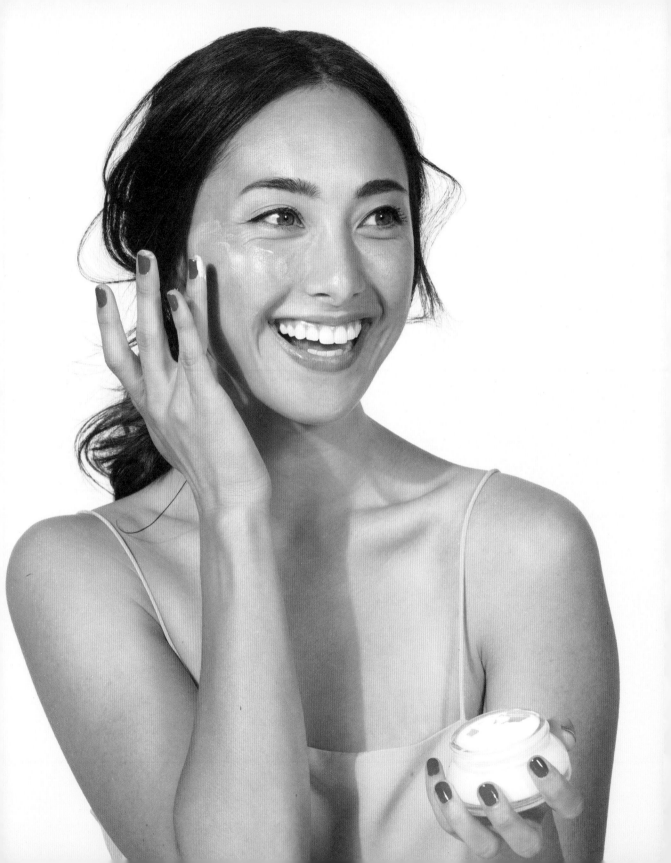

daily skincare routine

Your skin isn't the same every day. It varies and your skincare should, too. Here's a basic skincare routine that works on most people. Be open and customize as needed based on your personal skin needs.

CLEANSE

Start your day cleansing your skin with your regular cleanser. At night use a regular cleanser to get rid of makeup and dirt. Don't skip this step! If you wear eye makeup, you may also need to use an eye makeup remover applied with a cotton pad before you cleanse.

LAYER

For great skin, the secret is to layer different hydrating products one by one, taking a minute to let each one sink in. Your skin will react differently to each product—plumping with a hydrating cream, smoothing with a lotion, calming with a cream. Products can work in tandem to create beautiful skin.

IN THE MORNING, start with your sunscreen (look for SPF 15 or above). Combination products that pair SPF with makeup or moisturizer are great if you are on the go. Tap eye cream underneath your eyes. Then layer a light hydrating moisturizer on top before applying your makeup. You don't want to your skin to be overly moisturized because makeup will just slide off. (Save more intensive creams for nighttime.) On dry skin days, I begin with a face oil before the SPF, let it absorb, and then layer a richer cream moisturizer (or balm if skin is really dry or I'm on a plane). To create the look of dewy skin when my skin is anything but, I pat another layer of oil high on my cheeks.

AT NIGHT after cleansing and toning, begin with your serum to rejuvenate, then layer a much thicker balm or an oil and moisturizer. If you wake up to soft, dewy skin, then you've gotten the mix right. If your skin is parched, you need a new combination.

CUSTOMIZE

To customize your skincare even more, try mixing moisturizers or serums with your makeup. You can take your face oil and mix it with your moisturizer to create a light yet hydrating product. Add some foundation for a custom tinted moisturizer. Mix serum and a balm for intensive hydration, and add a few drops of gel bronzer to get a really fresh, healthy glow.

get glowing skin

A SKIN GURU WEIGHS IN

Mila Moursi is one of the top Hollywood skin gurus, with devoted clients including Sandra Bullock and Jennifer Aniston. She has her own product line and outpost, Mila Moursi Advanced Skin Care and Mila Moursi Skin Care Institute and Day Spa. We share similar philosophies on beauty: we both believe that looking gorgeous is about much more than products. Here are her go-to tips for incredible skin.

LIFESTYLE: Beauty starts from inside, that's for sure. Live a full life, but remember that moderation is key with everything. Maintain a lifestyle where you eat well, hydrate sufficiently, breathe deeply, exercise often, sleep soundly, and meditate daily.

DIGESTION: Chew your food well and eat slowly. Taking care of your digestion will help your skin. Take a tablespoon of bran flakes every night to help cleanse your digestive tract. If you are allergic to bran, take probiotics. Avoid inflammatory food such as processed foods and sugars, as they will directly affect skin texture and condition as well as your overall health.

HYDRATION: Drink eight to ten glasses of water a day, but not more than that, as too much could lead to the loss of some essential minerals. If possible, drink alkaline water or add fresh lemon, as that helps your system detox and will hydrate you quicker.

CLEANSE: Daily facial cleansing is a must for removing toxins and oils. Good cleansing leads to good oxygenation. When cleansing your face, use quick, fast, circular movements with your fingers and then remove the cleanser with a warm washcloth. Follow with a toner to complete the cleansing process.

DRY BRUSH: Using a dry body brush on the skin from head to toe daily takes only a few minutes and improves circulation, exfoliates dead skin cells, promotes lymphatic drainage, and helps remove toxins.

SUNSHINE: If possible, spend some time outdoors every day. A little bit of sun is not your enemy; sun is healthy for bones and skin, as it delivers essential vitamin D and is also a mood elevator. Apply the appropriate SPF and moderate your sun exposure depending on your skin type, family history, age, and any health concerns.

DON'T MIX BRANDS: Sometimes different brands have active ingredients that aren't compatible with each other.

GIVE PRODUCTS A CHANCE: It takes time for products to create change. If they are not giving you results after two months, then you can try something else, but it takes time to see results.

FACIALS AND FACIAL MASSAGE: Regular facial treatments can make you look younger very quickly. At home you can also improve your skin with massage. Daily massage promotes blood flow and oxygenation for vibrant skin. Wake up your skin with the tapotement technique, which is a light fluttering of your fingers along the skin (as if you are playing piano). For best results, do this after you apply your serum to further activate the active ingredients in the product. To incorporate a gentle massaging stroke technique into your skincare routine, apply a cream, oil, or balm, and then start at the center of your face, moving upward to the sides of the face with overlapping strokes using flat hands. To massage the neck, apply cream, balm, or oil to the skin. Then use upward strokes from the clavicle to the jawline. Continue along the jawline from the chin to the ear with a sliding, lifting stroke. Repeat ten strokes for each side of the neck and face. After, you can also pinch along the jawline to bring more blood flow to the lower face area.

spa treatments

A FACIALIST WEIGHS IN

Facials used to be all about massage and products. Now, there are dozens of excellent spa technologies used to make your skin look its best. Facialist Tracie Martyn has a devoted following of clients who rely on her to give them cutting-edge face and body treatments. "I use a lot of advanced technology in my treatments, including different colored LED lights depending on the needs of my clients (red for energizing and lifting, amber for wrinkles, and blue for acne), as well as my proprietary Resculptor, an amazing beauty machine that channels a mild current onto the skin to help firm, lift, and contour the face," explains Martyn. "However, I still use my hands, and I feel that the human touch with a healing intention sets my facials apart from the 'coldness' often associated with dermatological treatments."

To understand all of the technologies used in today's facials, Martyn breaks it down:

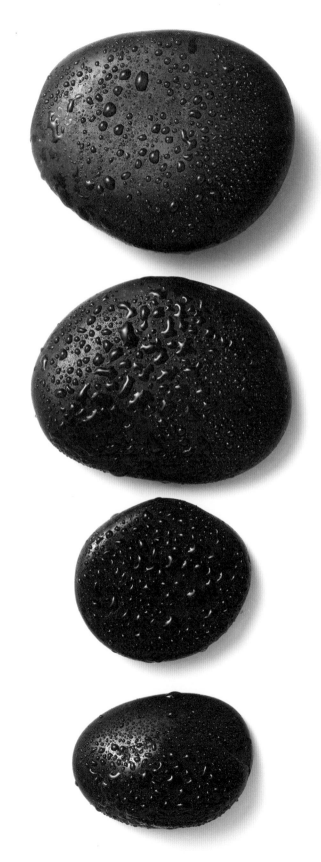

LED THERAPY

Light-emitting diode (LED) therapy is painless, noninvasive, and—unlike lasers—requires no recovery time. It can even improve your mood. (Studies with red light have shown improvements in seasonal affective disorder.)

Biologists have found that cells exposed to red light from LEDs regenerate 150 to 200 percent faster. The light increases energy inside cells (in the form of adenosine triphosphate, or ATP), which speeds up the healing process.

For those looking to reduce the signs of aging, red light and amber light are the best options. Red LED therapy can improve the appearance of skin, making it look younger, smoother, firmer, and healthier, and can also speed up the recovery process and help reduce inflammation after a more invasive aesthetic procedure. Pulsating amber light has been shown to reduce wrinkles and stop the stress enzymes known as matrix metalloproteinases (MMPs), which can cause wrinkles, lack of elasticity, and sun damage such as brown spots and other pigmentation. It takes less than a minute to "charge" the skin cells, getting them to produce more collagen and elastin, resulting in glowing, smoother skin over time.

Studies show that blue LED light has the remarkable ability to kill acne-causing bacteria, including *Propionibacterium acnes*. While results vary depending on a person's health, diet, skin color, skin tone, age, and lifestyle, profound changes and cumulative results are usually achieved in a series of six to eight treatments. Combining the blue light known for killing acne bacteria with the regenerative red light therapy creates a very effective synergy.

MICROCURRENTS

When used correctly, high-tech equipment powered by particular microcurrents, like the Resculptor, can lift, firm, and contour the jawline and the cheekbones and reduce puffiness and darkness in the eye area. There are great synergies between light and current, as both energize the treated area by stimulating the skin, resulting in younger-looking, smoother, and firmer face and body.

MICRODERMABRASION

Microdermabrasion is basically an exfoliation and skin rejuvenation procedure that leaves skin looking softer and brighter by removing an outer layer of dead skin cells and grime through a wand or by blasting aluminum oxide crystals onto the skin.

OXYGEN

Oxygen has regenerative powers to help your skin gain elasticity and glow and a have a healthy tone. Oxygen treatments, which apply oxygen to the face through a wand and serums, are gaining popularity and can smooth, tighten, and even out skin.

solutions for common skin issues

A NUTRITIONIST AND A DERMATOLOGIST WEIGH IN

People are often surprised to learn that what they eat can affect their skin. But common issues from acne to eczema can actually be triggered by different foods. When you are having a skin issue, the answer could be as simple as eating or avoiding certain foods, or it might need a prescription-strength solution. Here, nutritionist and founder of Foodtrainers Lauren Slayton and dermatologist Dr. Rosemarie Ingleton share their advice on six common skin issues.

acne

NUTRITIONIST'S ADVICE: Major acne triggers are dairy and sugary foods that cause blood sugar to spike. For clients with acne issues, I recommend ingesting maca, cinnamon, and apple cider vinegar daily. Maca is a hormone balancer, and cinnamon and apple cider vinegar have blood sugar benefits. Mix one large spoonful of apple cider vinegar in a glass of water and drink before breakfast or dinner. To work cinnamon or maca into your diet, try adding a dash of Ceylon cinnamon and one small spoonful of organic maca powder into a smoothie.

DERMATOLOGIST'S ADVICE: If you have a flare-up of acne, it's important to switch your moisturizer and cleansers to oil-free and non-comedogenic versions. Then add in products that will target the bacteria that causes acne. Start with over-the-counter versions that contain salicylic acid and apply to affected areas. If those don't clear up your skin, your dermatologist can give you a prescription based on exactly what kind of acne you have. Depending on your skin, benzoyl peroxide, retinoids, isotretinoin, or sulfur-based products are common solutions.

eczema and rosacea

NUTRITIONIST'S ADVICE: Vegetarian sources of protein such as beans and lentils, along with oolong tea, have been proven to help eczema sufferers. A dairy-free diet is helpful for both eczema and rosacea. Probiotics found in yogurt and supplements can also help both skin issues. With supplements, look for one with multiple types of probiotics (such as bifido, acidophilus, and rhamnosus) at a dose of 30 billion CFUs or more. Fermented veggies such as kimchi and fermented carrots are another powerful source of probiotics.

DERMATOLOGIST'S ADVICE: For eczema, avoid body washes, soaps, and lotions with fragrance, as they can aggravate it. Use rich moisturizers that have ceramides for intense hydration and soothing. For serious cases, add prescription topical steroids, and the situation should resolve in 10 to 14 days.

With rosacea, flare-ups generally occur after triggers like spicy foods, red wine, too much sun, or cold temperatures. Rosacea is a lifelong condition that can be managed by using a gentle cleanser, applying sunscreen, and avoiding known triggers.

dark circles

NUTRITIONIST'S ADVICE: Oftentimes dark circles or puffiness are caused by allergies. There are natural antihistamines such as quercetin, a flavonoid, that can help with these symptoms. Good sources of quercetin include dark berries such as blackberries and blueberries and green tea, and you can also buy quercetin supplements. For best results, ingest berries, green tea, or the supplements one or two times a day.

DERMATOLOGIST'S ADVICE: Dark circles are caused by many different factors, including allergies, congestion, genetics, and aging. Depending on the source, a cosmetic dermatologist can help with the right treatment, which could include lasers, antihistamines, fillers, and creams with green tea and vitamin K.

wrinkles

NUTRITIONIST'S ADVICE: Some foods can actually boost collagen and therefore minimize wrinkles. I love bone broth and gelatin for a dietary collagen boost. In terms of non-animal products, vitamin C is also an anti-aging winner, both taken as a supplement and applied to the skin as a serum.

DERMATOLOGIST'S ADVICE: The sun is the biggest wrinkle culprit, so use sunscreen (SPF 30 or higher) daily and wear hats in strong sun. Avoid tanning and sunbathing. Products that contain retinoids and fruit acids help promote skin renewal and soften lines; apply these topical antioxidants daily to help heal and correct environmental aging.

dry skin

NUTRITIONIST'S ADVICE: Dry skin can be a sign that more vitamin A is needed. Sweet potatoes and leafy greens such as spinach and kale are great dietary sources of vitamin A. Zinc helps enhance the effects of vitamin A. Shellfish, carrots, and pumpkin seeds are also excellent sources of the nutrient.

DERMATOLOGIST'S ADVICE: To combat dry skin, you have to hydrate inside and out. Drink at least eight glasses of water a day. With topical products, make sure everything you use—cleanser, soap, serums, and lotions—are all formulated to be extra hydrating. Look for formulas with glycerin. Oils are also extremely moisturizing. The best ones for dry skin are sesame oil, olive oil, macadamia nut oil, and almond oil; you can apply them directly to the skin daily.

home spa

By now you know about the powerful effects of beauty foods on your health, skin, and overall glow. But the items in your pantry and fridge can also be applied directly to hair and skin for even more radiance. From masks to scrubs to moisturizers, here are my favorite kitchen beauty treatments.

HAIR CONDITIONERS

AVOCADO, OLIVE, OR COCONUT OIL: All three of these will give your hair an intense boost of moisture. Olive oil is the most intense, followed by coconut oil. Avocado is lighter but still hydrating. Just shampoo your hair, squeeze out excess water, and coat your hair with the oil. Tie up your hair with an elastic and let the oil soak in for 15 minutes, then rinse it out. I recommend doing an oil treatment once a week. If you have oily hair or an oily scalp, coat only the ends.

HAIR SHINE BOOST

APPLE CIDER VINEGAR: Shampoos and conditioners can leave build up over time, leaving hair lifeless and flat. To bring your hair back to health, rinse with one cup of apple cider vinegar after shampooing. Rinse with water and then condition as usual. Do this when you feel your hair looking dull, then repeat once a month.

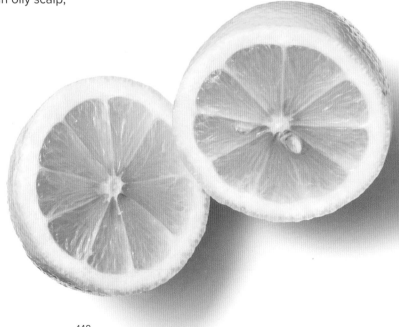

ACNE FIGHTERS

LEMON: This works as a great astringent for oily skin. Just dip a cotton ball into fresh-squeezed lemon juice and apply to your T-zone or anywhere skin is clogged and oily. You can also use lemon juice as a spot treatment for pimples.

BODY SCRUBS

I personally love a deep, strong exfoliator for some of the rougher areas on my body, and my quest for this ended in my kitchen. While cleaning out my gadget drawer, I found an unused potato scrubber glove that actually worked wonders. It now lives in my shower and I use it regularly on my legs and feet. This is definitely not for everyone, but it shows how a little creativity is sometimes all that is needed when it comes to beauty.

BROWN SUGAR AND OLIVE OIL: This gentle body scrub works to exfoliate and moisturize if you apply it to your body before a shower, then rinse off. Mix two parts olive oil with one part brown sugar. Your skin will be so hydrated you won't have to apply moisturizer afterward.

SEA SALT, LEMON JUICE, AND OLIVE OIL: For a more intense scrub, combine two parts olive oil with one part sea salt and one part lemon juice. The lemon acts as an astringent, while the sea salt provides a more vigorous scrub and the olive oil hydrates. Use before or during a shower to reveal fresh skin.

LIP SCRUB

HONEY WITH BROWN SUGAR: Mix two parts honey with one part brown sugar for a sweet and exfoliating lip scrub. Rub gently in a circular motion until sugar is dissolved. Wipe off any excess with a tissue, and follow with lip balm.

MAKEUP REMOVERS

OLIVE OIL, COCONUT OIL, JOJOBA OIL: Pretty much any natural oil will work to effortlessly remove makeup plus add a hydrating boost to skin. Just apply oils to a cotton pad and sweep across face to lift off makeup.

MOISTURIZERS

CUSTOM OIL BLENDS: I created my dream face oil for my brand more than ten years ago with vitamin E and sesame, sweet almond, olive, and jojoba oils, plus neroli, patchouli, lavender, and sandalwood for fragrance. I also use a lot of oils from my kitchen on my face and body. Try customizing your own. Pair any oils you love (olive, coconut, grapeseed, and avocado oils are all very hydrating), then mix with a few drops of essential oils for scent (my favorites are neroli and orange essence). Place in a pretty glass bottle and you have your own custom hydrating miracle oil.

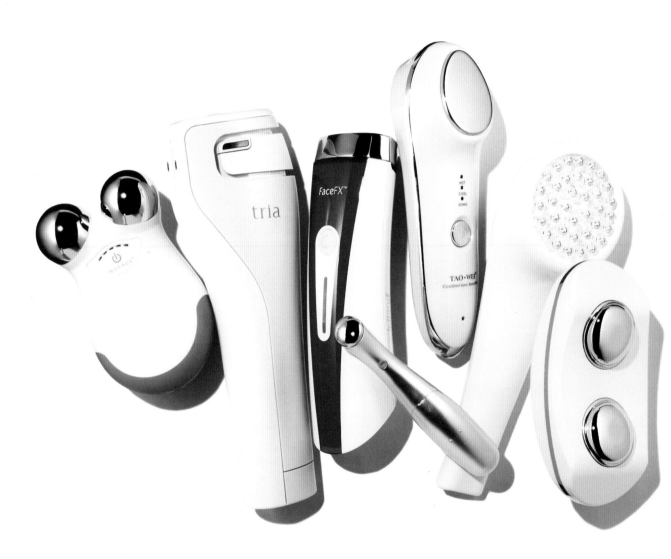

6

Beauty Break-throughs

*T*here are new beauty breakthroughs emerging every day. What I'm most excited about is the painless, noninvasive laser procedures that tone, firm, and even out skin without altering your looks. They promise fresher, clearer, plumper skin and are also used for fat reduction and body smoothing.

This is a big change from twenty years ago, when, if you wanted tighter, younger-looking skin, your only option was surgery. Even ten years ago, the choices were focused almost solely on the quest for the fountain of youth. It was either filler or Botox, which in my experience are not great choices if you want to have a natural look.

Today you can tackle anything from sunspots to sagging skin to acne to stubborn fat—in minutes!—without the scars, pain, or long recovery times of surgery. You can even do some of these procedures on your own, thanks to new at-home technologies.

Like so many women, I am fascinated by what's new, but it takes time and experience to discover what really works and what doesn't. I turned to a team of top doctors to highlight some of the most effective treatment options available. My aesthetic has always been about the glow that comes from a healthy lifestyle and great attitude. I definitely believe less is more here, so I've spotlighted treatments that don't alter the face to make you look different, but rather refresh and restore your natural beauty.

WHAT REALLY WORKS

I love lines on a face, I really do. They add expression, character, and life, and they look natural. That's why I am excited by lasers and radiofrequency devices. They increase collagen and eliminate sunspots (which are the first sign of aging), but they don't alter your face or freeze lines the way fillers do.

I first tried Botox in my 40s. I didn't like it. I couldn't move my forehead. I looked altered. Once, it gave me a pointy eyebrow, and another time it caused one eye to droop. It definitely wasn't for me. I have done lasers and loved them—I've zapped off sunspots and, after a little bit of pain, the treatment works wonders. I've also had Ultherapy, an ultrasound treatment, and Thermage, a radio-frequency treatment, both of which were more than mildly painful, but also super-effective in producing collagen, lifting, and tightening. There are new lasers that are far less painful and work quite well. TriPollar technology is great for tightening the neck and jaw, and it seems to start working halfway through the treatment. The treatment I most recommend is laser hair removal. It is totally life-changing. However, it was also very time-consuming (it required several treatments over months) and not cheap, unfortunately.

There are also less expensive home options available. I love NuFACE, a home microcurrent treatment you can buy online. It helps firm your neck and tighten and lift the skin. The effects aren't permanent, but you see results right away. They cost as much as many spas charge for one or two microcurrent treatments, so there is cost savings over time.

My rule of thumb is to stick with procedures that make me look fresher and lifted—but most importantly still like me. With plastic surgery or even fillers, you can alter your face to such an extreme you no longer look like yourself, and there's no going back if you don't like it.

transforming treatments

There's an incredible range of treatments available. To help you navigate through all the hype, here's the breakdown of the most effective treatments and the scoop on each one. Prices for treatments vary depending on where you live, and what's expensive to one woman might not seem so to another. The guide to pricing is as follows: moderate = low hundreds; expensive = high hundreds; and very expensive = thousands.

microcurrents

WHAT IT DOES: This device delivers tiny electrical currents to the skin that cause muscles to contract, immediately tightening the skin.

WHO IT'S BEST FOR: Those who want an immediately noticeable lifted and sculpted look. The treatment is particularly great for jawlines and cheekbones. However, it is a temporary lifting, although many facialists claim that regular appointments (weekly or monthly depending on the patient) will keep skin lifted.

TIME REQUIRED: 5 to 15 minutes. Many facialists do microcurrents as part of a facial. You can also do it yourself with an at-home microcurrent machine.

PAIN FACTOR: None. Expect a little skin tingling during the treatment.

COST: Moderate at a spa. At-home devices like NuFACE are a moderate investment but can be used for multiple home treatments.

THE DOCTOR SAYS: "Overall there are not many solid clinical studies evaluating the anti-aging effects of these treatments," explains dermatologist Dr. Sejal Shah. "However, some people may find that these treatments work because their facial muscles respond immediately by contracting, so there is some validity to the effects of microcurrents."

laser hair removal

WHAT IT DOES: A light laser is aimed at hair follicles to prevent hair growth. It can be done anywhere you have unwanted hair; legs, bikini line, back, and underarms are popular choices.

WHO IT'S BEST FOR: People who are tired of the repetition and hassle of shaving and waxing and want a more permanent hair-removal solution. It's more effective on patients with darker hair; it won't work as well on blondes.

TIME REQUIRED: It takes several sessions to remove the hair—on average, five sessions spaced six weeks apart—however, that number varies depending on the patient and area treated. Touchups will be needed if hair starts to grow back (which it may).

PAIN FACTOR: Patients lie down and a technician zaps hair follicles with a laser. Each blast feels like a rubber band snapping against the skin. It can be painful. Discomfort can be minimized by taking ibuprofen prior to the treatment.

RECOVERY: You may experience some mild redness and burning for a few hours. After each session, hair will grow back thinner and thinner until it's gone.

COST: Moderate to expensive depending on how many sessions are needed.

THE DOCTOR SAYS: "Unlike shaving or waxing, laser hair removal generally does not cause ingrown hairs. And unlike depilatory creams, it does not contain chemicals that can irritate the skin or cause reactions. These methods can also be tough on sensitive areas, compared to laser hair removal," explains Dr. Shah. "There is a risk of burn if not performed properly; therefore, it is important to see someone who is well-trained and experienced so they use the correct laser for your skin type."

peels

If you want to reveal new skin and tackle common skin issues such as acne without the high cost of lasers, then peels are for you. While the procedure has been around for fifty years, the current versions cause less irritation and redness than their predecessors while still revealing more radiant skin. Make sure, however, that you opt for a mild to medium peel rather than a more aggressive one that carries risks and can leave your skin irritated, red, and painful for days. The intensity scale is based on the percentage of acid in the peel. Note that the peels you get at home are the mildest (and honestly least effective). Spa peels are also usually on the mild side, too. The most effective mild to medium peels can be found at your dermatologist's office.

WHAT IT IS: An acid solution applied topically that causes skin to peel five days after treatment to reveal a new layer of skin and minimize wrinkles, acne, and skin discoloration. Peels often have the consistency of a gel or gooey liquid.

WHO IT'S BEST FOR: Those looking for a treatment to clear up their skin without the higher price tag of laser treatments.

TIME REQUIRED: After it is applied to the skin, the peel takes 5 to 15 minutes to complete. The gel is easy to rinse off and then you're ready to go. The results aren't immediate, but about five days after the peel, skin will be flaky and then peel off, revealing the younger skin. To keep up results, do a peel two or three times a year.

PAIN FACTOR: Always go with a mild to medium peel, as you can have amazing results without the extreme redness or pain associated with higher concentrations (although you may have some mild redness). Some mild stinging could occur during the treatment, but otherwise the peel should be painless.

RECOVERY: This will depend on the strength of the peel and your sensitivity, but with a mild to medium peel you should have some mild redness the first day and flaking after five days. After a week you will see clearer, tighter skin.

COST: Moderate.

THE DOCTOR SAYS: "One of my favorite peels is the Vitalize Peel from SkinMedica," says holistic plastic surgeon Dr. Shirley Madhere. "It's a combination of three acids: alpha hydroxy, beta hydroxy, and a retinoic to soften fine lines, stimulate collagen, improve hyperpigmentation, and brighten skin. It works for women of all skin tones, and as it is a mild- to medium-depth peel, it can be applied to most people without serious redness."

radio frequency

Radio frequency devices tone and tighten the skin, and results can last for up to two years. A standard radio frequency device is paired with a coupling emulsion or gel during application to deliver radio frequency waves below the surface of the skin. Some devices pair RF with micro-needling, which puncture the skin to deliver a more intense treatment.

TRIPOLLAR

WHAT IT DOES: This device reduces the appearance of fine lines and lifts and tightens skin.

WHO IT'S BEST FOR: People with mild to moderate skin sagging on their face and/or neck.

TIME REQUIRED: The treatment takes 20 minutes. You will start to see results after two weeks, and the treatment will keep working for up to six months. Expect to do two to four treatments performed about a month apart, but results are visible after the first treatment.

PAIN FACTOR: None. This treatment uses a non-ablative (non-puncturing) device so it doesn't penetrate the skin, making it painless.

RECOVERY: None. Possibility of mild redness on the day of the treatment.

COST: Expensive.

THE DOCTOR SAYS: "TriPollar uses three times the amount of radio frequency as other popular radio frequency treatments, so it's faster and more effective, without the pain. It's really the future of non-invasive skin technologies," says derma-tologist Dr. Macrene Alexiades.

PROFOUND

WHAT IT DOES: This needle-based radio frequency treatment creates new elastin, collagen, and hyaluronic acid (and is the only device to help skin create all three). It can lift and contour sagging jawlines as well as restore volume to skin.

WHO IT'S BEST FOR: People with moderate to severe sagging.

TIME REQUIRED: The treatment takes about an hour and a half. You see results in about a month, and the treatment keeps working for about a year.

PAIN FACTOR: Thanks to hair-fine needles paired with topical lidocaine, discomfort is minimal to none.

RECOVERY: Expect swelling and bruising for five to seven days.

COST: Expensive.

THE DOCTOR SAYS: "Profound is the closest we have gotten to a surgical facelift with nonsurgical methods," explains Dr. Alexiades.

lasers

Lasers are the magic wands of the beauty world. They can improve the appearance of acne, sunspots, wrinkles, minor scars, and other irregularities, leaving your skin smoother, clearer, and glowing. In general, a non-ablative laser treatment is the milder choice, heating up the targeted tissue without actually destroying it. If you are trying lasers for the first time, a non-ablative laser should be where you start.

An ablative laser goes deeper and requires fewer treatments, but it can mean a week of downtime while your skin is swollen and red. Ablative laser may be the route for you if you don't want to endure multiple treatments and can tolerate the recovery and downtime.

CLEAR + BRILLIANT

WHAT IT DOES: This is a gentle fractional laser treatment that stimulates collagen production. "A fractional laser applies laser energy to small areas, or fractions, of the skin at a time," explains Dr. Shah. "The laser targets and treats intensively within the treatment zone while the surrounding, untreated tissue remains intact. This results in a faster healing process than if all tissue in the area was exposed to the laser, as it is [with] a fully ablative laser. Fractional lasers bridge the gap between ablative and non-ablative lasers and, depending on the laser and what is being treated and the individual, you can potentially achieve ablative-like results without the downtime." The device improves skin texture and tone and increases radiance. It also reduces the appearance of pores for clearer, healthier-looking skin.

WHO IT'S BEST FOR: Those who want smaller pores and clearer skin, or to tackle the early signs of aging. Someone with deep wrinkles or acne scars should go with a more intense option. Clear + Brilliant is safe for all skin types, including darker skin.

TIME REQUIRED: About 30 minutes for the numbing cream application and 20 minutes for the laser treatment. Expect four to six sessions spaced a few weeks apart. "Almost everyone has some improvement after one treatment," says Dr. Shah.

PAIN FACTOR: As long as a topical numbing agent is applied beforehand, the treatment should be painless.

RECOVERY: For the first 12 to 24 hours, expect pink or red skin, which can be reduced with ice or a calming serum or mask. Your skin may have a sandpaper-like texture for up to a week after the treatment. You may experience increased skin sensitivity and/or itching for the first few days.

COST: Moderate to expensive per treatment.

THE DOCTOR SAYS: Clear + Brilliant, or "Baby Fraxel, as I like to call it, is one of my favorite laser treatments," says Dr. Shah. "It is my go-to treatment for anyone who is looking to improve skin texture and tone and boost radiance, or even maintain their skin's appearance, with no downtime." Note that it is a maintenance treatment, not a corrective treatment. "There can be improvement in fine lines, skin texture, and pigmentation after a series of treatments, but it does not stop the aging process, so over time if the treatment is not maintained, the skin issues can reappear or new lines or textural and pigment changes can occur," says Dr. Shah. "I have had some patients who have seen long-term improvement of pigment issues like freckles or melasma, but since UV radiation plays a role in the development of these conditions, new spots can [appear] over time."

FRAXEL RESTORE DUAL

WHAT IT DOES: This fractional laser stimulates collagen and rejuvenates skin cells below the surface by causing micro-injuries to the skin. The laser targets fine lines, wrinkles, sun damage, and scarring.

WHO IT'S BEST FOR: For those with noticeable sun damage, wrinkles, or age spots and who want to significantly improve skin issues without the pain or longer recovery of a more aggressive laser like the Fraxel Repair.

TIME REQUIRED: Generally patients need three to five sessions spaced a month apart. The entire face takes around 20 minutes to do, after applying a numbing cream for 60 minutes prior. If your concern is brown spots/age spots, you may see significant improvement after just one treatment.

PAIN FACTOR: Some patients find the treatment uncomfortable, noting a burning sensation that can last for 24 hours after the procedure.

RECOVERY: Expect one to three days of redness and puffiness. Your skin may have a sunburned appearance, and there may be some peeling in the first week, especially if you have a lot of brown spots or age spots.

COST: Very expensive.

THE DOCTOR SAYS: "Fraxel is a proven laser technology that can help reverse the visible signs of aging and textural abnormalities," explains Dr. Shah. "It really gives you a more natural-appearing, youthful, radiant look without entirely changing your appearance. It's you, just better."

fat reduction technology

For years the only way to get rid of excess fat (that is, fat that does not go away through diet and exercise) was through liposuction or laser liposuction. Both procedures have serious recovery time and cause significant scarring. Today there are several nonsurgical options for targeting stubborn fat cells. Kybella is an injectable for underneath the chin, while CoolSculpting uses controlled cooling through a wand to target and kill fat cells. The procedure literally freezes fat during a session. For up to a month afterward, the body slowly eliminates those fat cells.

COOLSCULPTING

WHAT IT DOES: A device freezes and destroys fat cells, promising a 20 to 25 percent reduction in fat thickness with each treatment.

WHO IT'S BEST FOR: People who have stubborn spots of fat on their thighs, hips, waist, or stomach that diet and exercise can't eliminate. The latest product, Cool-Mini, is designed specifically for reducing double chins. Note that this treatment won't work for patients who are obese.

TIME REQUIRED: The actual treatment takes from one to three hours depending on the size of the area treated. Expect to wait one to three months for the fat to dissipate and to see results. Most patients need at least two treatments.

PAIN FACTOR: There are no needles or surgery involved, but you may experience some discomfort as the fat is frozen with the wand. The fat hardens when it is frozen and is then massaged by your doctor or technician to break up the fat.

RECOVERY: None.

COST: Moderate to expensive. With at least two treatments needed, the costs add up.

THE DOCTOR SAYS: "CoolSculpting is really the frontrunner with fat reduction devices," explains Dr. Alexiades. "It is the most effective noninvasive fat-reducing technology on the market today that has the advantages of no scars, no downtime, and the best safety profile as compared to liposuction or other laser- and light-based fat treatments."

SCULPSURE

WHAT IT DOES: This wand treatment heats and destroys fat cells with a laser light.

WHO IT'S BEST FOR: People who have stubborn spots of excess fat that diet and exercise can't eliminate on their thighs, hips, waist, or stomach. The treatment won't work for obese patients.

TIME REQUIRED: The actual treatment takes from one to two hours depending on the size of the area treated. Expect to wait six to twelve weeks for the fat to dissipate and to see results. Most patients need at least two treatments.

PAIN FACTOR: Minimal. There may be some discomfort during the procedure.

RECOVERY: Expect some minor swelling and soreness or tenderness of the treated area for the first week.

COST: Moderate to expensive.

THE DOCTOR SAYS: "The treatment is different from dieting, where you lose fat from within the fat cells but those cells still exist," explains plastic surgeon Dr. Lawrence Bass. "With SculpSure we are damaging the fat cells so they are eliminated completely."

KYBELLA

WHAT IT DOES: Known as Belkyra in certain overseas markets, this treatment involves injections of deoxycholic acid administered underneath the chin to eliminate fat cells. It is identical to the deoxycholic acid naturally produced by our bodies to help the body absorb fats.

WHO IT'S BEST FOR: Patients with mild to moderate fat under the chin. Patients who are obese or who have a neck that requires a lot of skin tightening should try other options.

TIME REQUIRED: The 30-minute treatment (15 for numbing, 15 for injections) involves dozens of small injections targeting the fat under the chin. Most patients average three treatments administered four to six weeks apart, but some will require six treatments. The results are permanent.

PAIN FACTOR: A topical numbing cream should be applied first. Patients will feel the prick of at least twenty injections and then possibly a burning sensation at the injection sites that can last a few minutes.

RECOVERY: Patients may experience some bruising, redness, and swelling that can last about a week (although occasionally longer) as the fat melts away. Some patients experience very obvious swelling (even larger than the original double chin), making this a procedure best done in colder months, when they can recover under a turtleneck.

COST: Very expensive.

THE DOCTOR SAYS: "Kybella is the first-ever injectable fat-dissolving substance that safely, reliably, and reproducibly eliminates fat under the chin quickly in the office with a very quick and easy recovery," explains Dr. Alexiades.

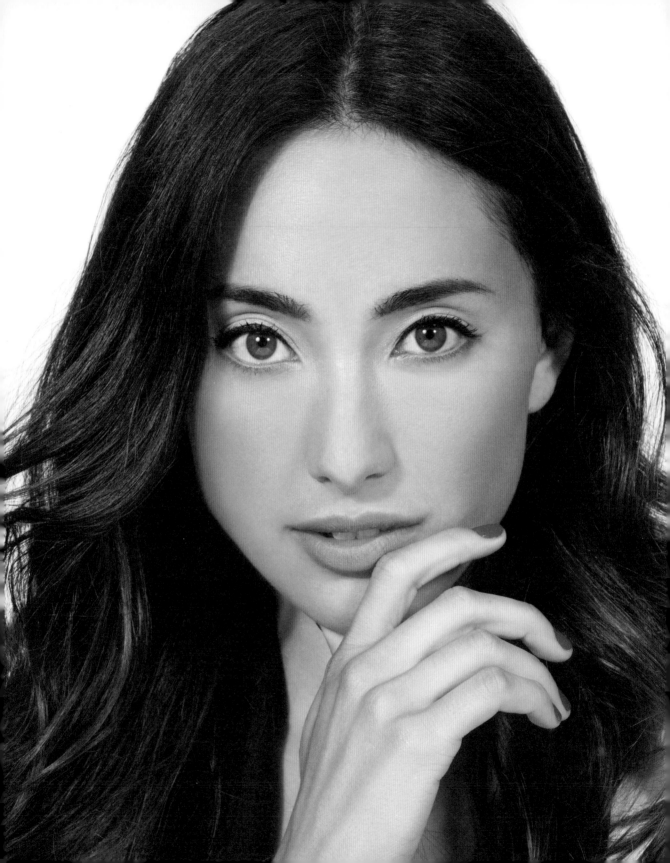

Basics for Beautiful Makeup

*I*t's amazing what even a little makeup can do. Concealer that hides a late night, liner that makes your eyes stand out, or blush that makes you look like you've just come in from a run. The right makeup can make you feel more beautiful and more confident.

Applying makeup can seem daunting (especially if you watch YouTube tutorials), but it doesn't have to be. If you know the tricks to making makeup look great, you can go on to make it your own. From picking the perfect foundation to covering up dark circles to mastering winged liner, there are easy ways to play up your strongest features.

Makeup isn't complicated. There are simple techniques and amazing products that make it easy to master. This chapter will start with the basics: how to pick the right products for you and how to apply them. Once you have the basics down, you'll be able to master all kinds of looks.

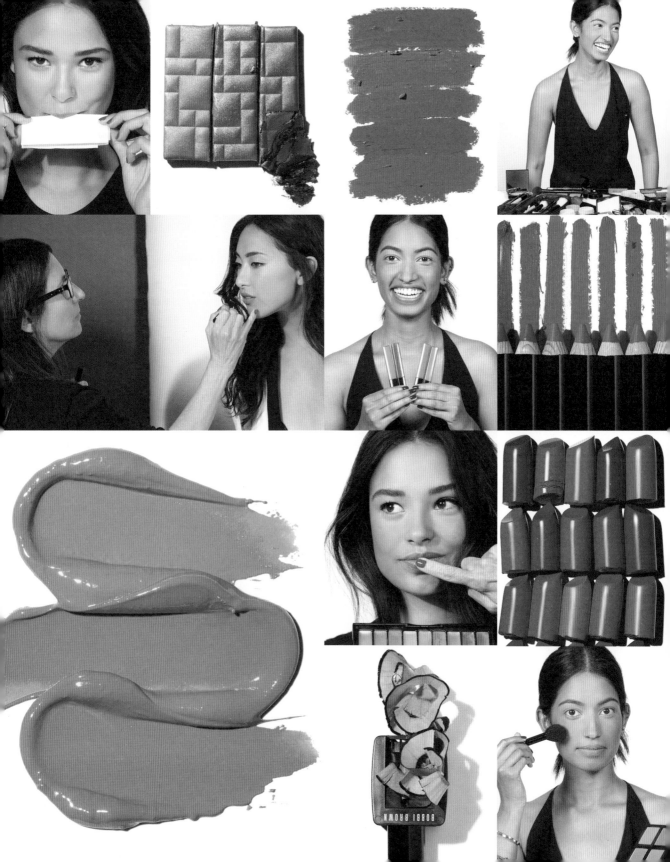

BOBBI BROWN

foundation

The right foundation blends seamlessly, evening out and enhancing your skin. To find the right match, start by deciding what formulas you need, from a lighter tinted moisturizer to an on-the-go stick. Choose full, medium, or light coverage next. Finally, make sure the color matches your skin exactly. Because skin color and type varies throughout the year, you will want to have a few different foundations on hand.

TYPES

TINTED MOISTURIZER: This moisturizer/foundation hybrid offers a light, translucent coverage.

BALM: Balm foundation is harder to find, but it combines intense moisture, a light tint, and a dewy finish. It's a good choice for mature or dry skin.

LIQUID: Liquid is the classic foundation formula and ranges from sheer to full coverage, glowy to matte. It can be applied with fingers, a brush, or a sponge.

STICK: Foundation sticks are made of creamy formulas that offer medium to full coverage in a convenient package. It's longer lasting, stands up to heat, and can also double as a concealer for face and body.

MINERAL: With no fragrance or chemicals, mineral foundation works well for sensitive or acne-prone skin. These are available in compact, loose powder, and liquid formulas and provide light to medium coverage.

POWDER: Set in a compact and applied with a brush, powder foundation offers medium coverage and is a good on-the-go choice.

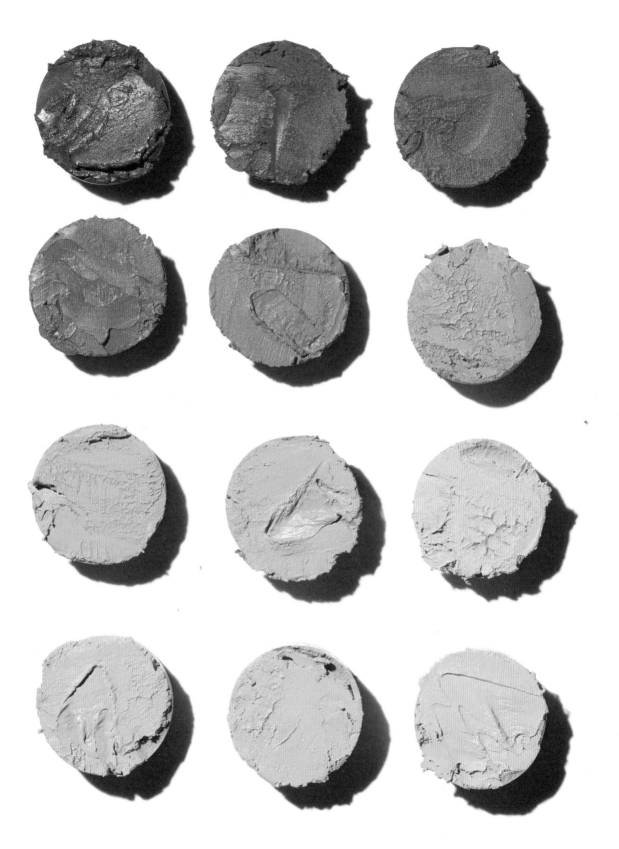

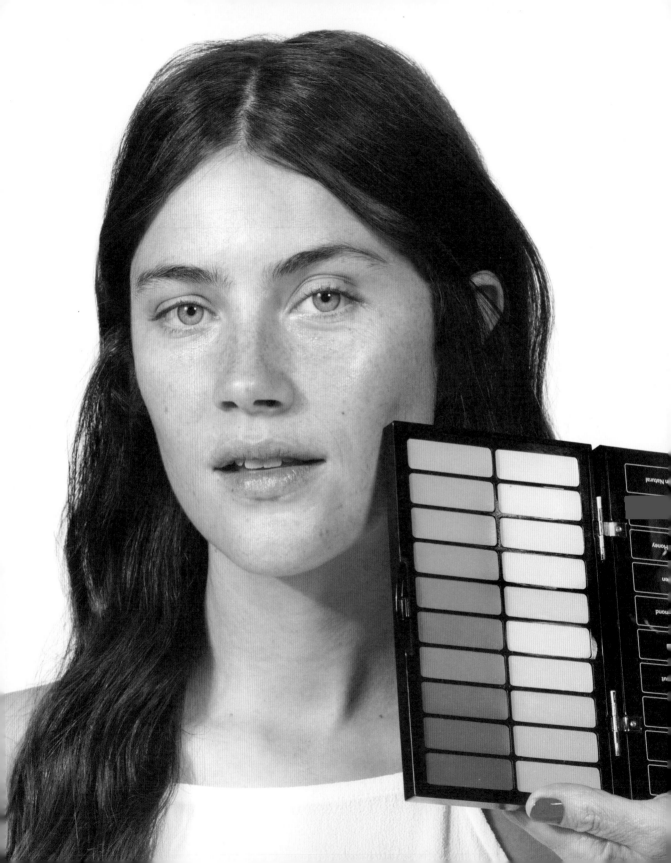

COVERAGE

SHEER/LIGHT: If you want a more natural appearance or are lucky enough to have great skin, go with a lighter formula. A tinted moisturizer offers the lightest coverage. Next is a sheer-to-light liquid formula. If your skin is very dry, look for a tinted cream or balm formula that offers hydrating benefits, too.

MEDIUM: Most foundation formulas are medium coverage, offering enough to hide imperfections but not so much that your makeup looks heavy. You'll find medium-coverage versions for powder, liquid, and stick foundations.

FULL: These types of foundations will fully cover your skin to eliminate the appearance of any imperfections or redness. For evening makeup or more of a Hollywood retro look, go with full coverage. You can find versions in powder, liquid, and stick forms.

FINISHES

Once you decide how much coverage you need, decide what you want the finish to look like, taking your skin type into account. Do you prefer a dewy or matte look? Do you need a foundation that also moisturizes or do you want one that controls shine? Luminous, hydrating, and moisturizing formulas will give you a glowy finish. A matte foundation will cut oil. Liquid formulas will give you coverage without looking dry or shiny. Oil-free formulas stay put during hot weather and are good options for people with oily skin.

COLOR MATCH

Unfortunately, you can't tell if a foundation color is right for you by just looking at the package or testing out a swipe on your hand or arm. You have to try it out on your face. On a makeup-free face, pick three shades close to your skin tone and apply them in two strips on your cheek. Check the colors in natural light; the color that blends in with your skin is the right one. If you are in between colors, go with the one that is slightly darker. If you have oily skin, go one shade lighter, as the oils in your skin can make your foundation change color. Most importantly, look for a yellow-toned foundation that will match the natural yellow undertones everyone has in their skin.

APPLICATION

I personally like to apply foundation with my fingers. It gives me more control of the product and I find that the warmth of my hands makes the product easier to apply. I also occasionally use a foundation brush, which gives a nice, even application.

corrector and concealer

These two products work together to tackle undereye darkness and discoloration. I always say that corrector and concealer are the secret of the universe. They brighten the undereye area and hide dark circles for an instant lift. For blemishes you need a targeted blemish concealer or a touchup pencil.

TYPES

CORRECTOR: Corrector is pink or peach-based, which neutralizes discoloration and brightens under your eyes. If you have light to medium skin, go with pink or bisque-toned corrector. Try peach corrector for warmer skin tones. Darker skin tones should look for dark bisque corrector. If your corrector looks too light or whitish, go with a darker shade. If your corrector looks too yellow, choose a lighter tone.

UNDEREYE CONCEALER: Undereye concealer lightens and hides darkness. Look for a yellow-based concealer for the undereye area. It should be one shade lighter than your skin tone. You want your concealer to last all day. Look for creamy formulas that blend easily into skin. (Many stick formulas do not.) Serum formulas offer intense coverage with a moisturizing boost that doesn't sink into fine lines.

BLEMISH CONCEALER: You never want to use your undereye concealer to cover a blemish because it is one shade lighter than your skin tone and will only highlight what you want to hide. Instead, choose a concealer designed for the face to spot cover any imperfections or redness. You can apply a face touchup stick directly to redness and blend with your fingers. Do this step before you apply foundation.

RETOUCHING PENCIL: For a quick, easy way to create even skin, reach for a retouching pencil that matches your skin tone. To cover dark spots and lighten shadows, choose a pencil one to two shades lighter than your skin tone. To cover redness, choose a shade that matches your skin tone. Apply directly to the area you want to lighten and blend with your fingers.

APPLICATION

Corrector and concealer are designed to be layered, with corrector placed first, followed by concealer. Use your fingers or a brush to apply, and then blend with a finger, tapping the product gently into your skin. Set concealer in place with a light dusting of yellow-toned powder. If you are very pale, a white powder may work better for you. If you have darker skin, try a peach-based powder. This should not be the same powder you apply to your whole face.

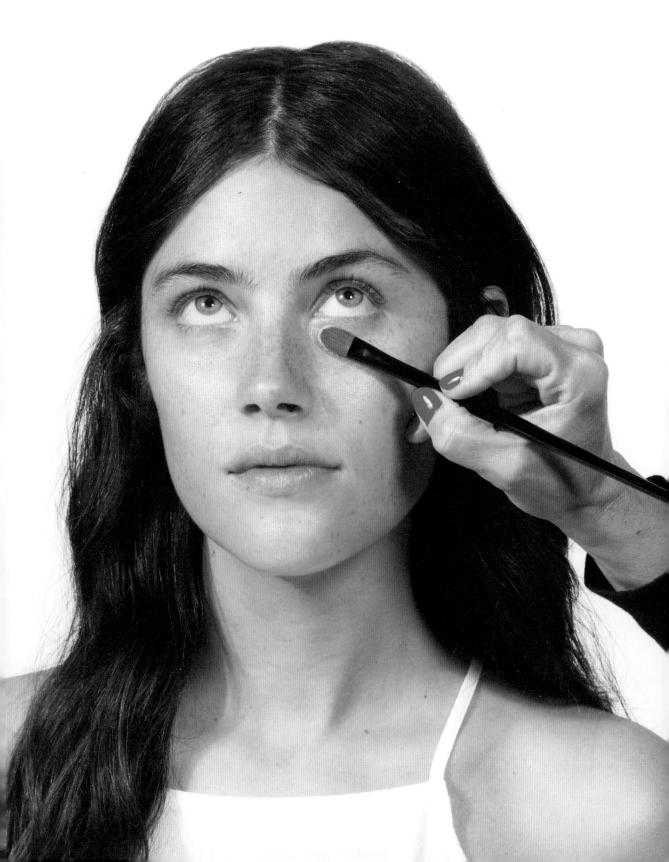

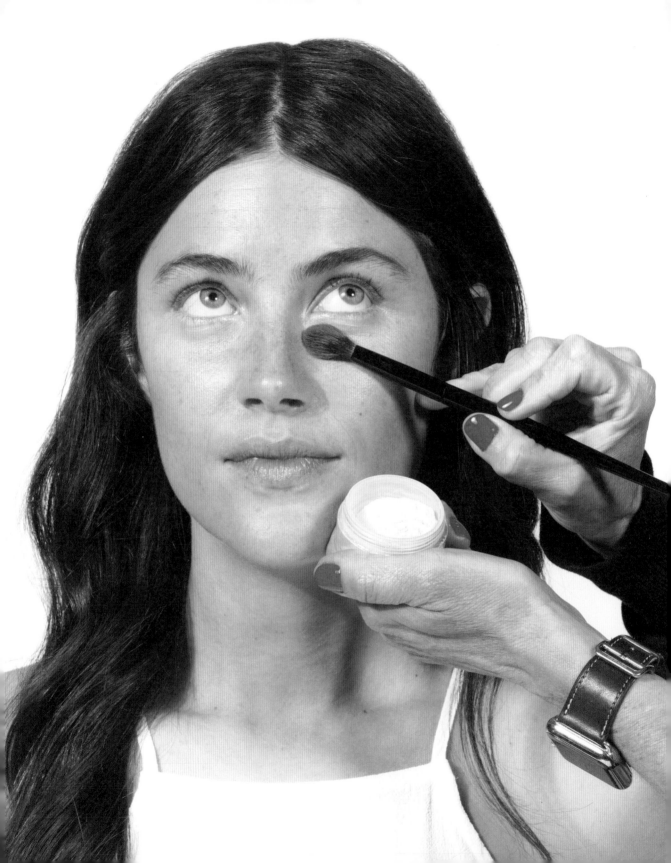

Powder cuts shine, evens out skin, and helps set your face makeup. It is the final step to make concealer and foundation last for hours. If you have very dry skin, skip this step altogether because powder will enhance dry areas.

powder

TYPES

There are two types of powder: pressed and loose. Pressed powder has a light finish and comes in a compact (often with a mirror), which makes it a great on-the-go option. Loose powder is denser and offers more complete coverage.

COLOR MATCH

For most people, a powder with a yellow undertone works to help cut redness and add warmth. Choose a shade that matches the color of your skin almost exactly. If you have very oily skin, powder can turn a darker shade, so go one shade lighter.

APPLICATION

You don't need to apply powder heavily. Just a light dusting to cut shine on the T-zone will work for most women. You can apply both pressed and loose powder with a brush for a light finish. If your skin is oily, use a powder puff and apply all over the face.

bronzer

———

Bronzer is a great way to look tan and healthy year-round. It's a product that everyone loves, including men. Some of my most popular bronzers are named after the guys I made them for, including actor Eric Stonestreet and radio personality Elvis Duran.

TYPES

Bronzer comes in liquid, gel, and powder formulas. A matte bronzer is the easiest to apply and works day or night. A bronzer with shimmer looks best at night. Gel formula gives a deeper color.

COLOR MATCH

Light brown bronzer with a hint of pink and coral is best for pale skin. Medium skin tones look good with a medium brownish pink or brownish coral. Women with dark skin should look for bronzer that is dark brown with blue or red undertones. Bronzers come in both shimmer and matte versions. If your bronzer looks too red, orange, or ashy, you have the wrong shade.

APPLICATION

To apply powder bronzer, use a large, flat brush on the apples of the cheeks. Dust over the nose, chin, and forehead—spots where the sun naturally hits the face. Apply to the neck as well.

To apply gel or cream bronzer, use your fingers or a sponge. Begin at the apples of the cheeks and blend outward toward the hairline. Make sure to blend. I always put a pop of brighter blush on top.

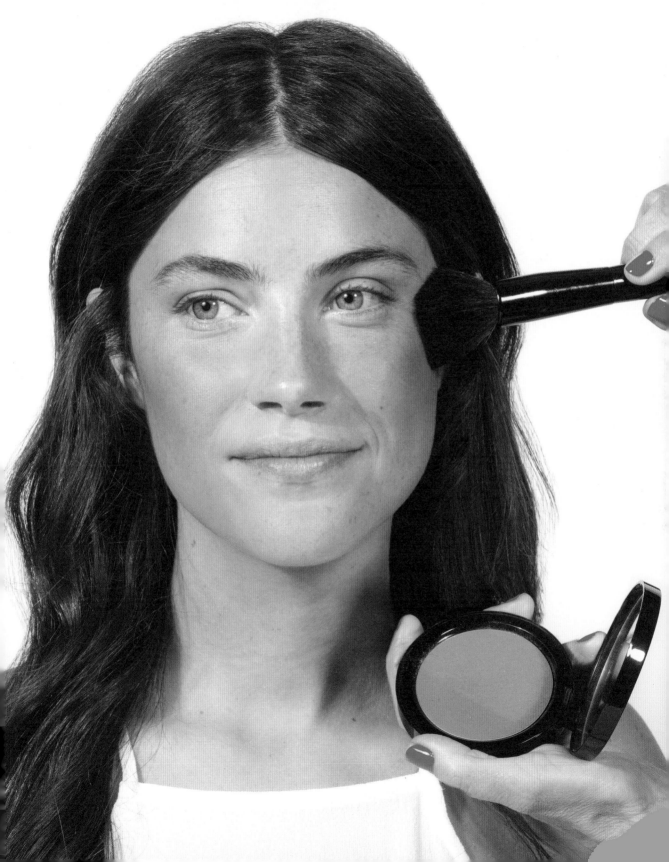

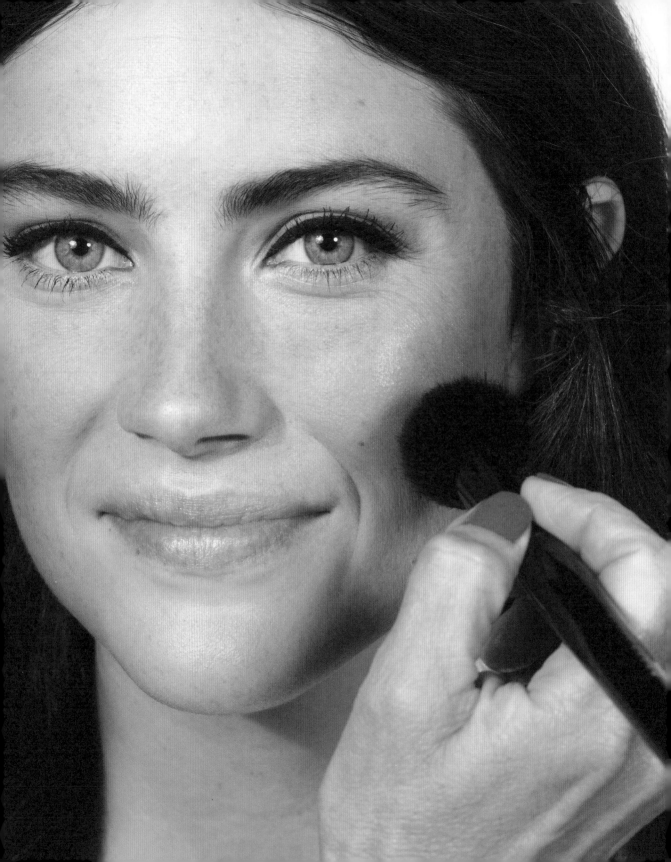

the perfect blush

Blush makes everyone look pretty. It warms up your complexion and brightens your face. A shade that matches the color your cheeks turn when they naturally flush is a good everyday choice. A pop of a brighter shade of pink or coral to layer over your everyday blush or bronzer will keep the color longer. You can use just a brighter blush for evening.

TYPES

Blush is available in powder, cream, or gel formulas. Powder is the easiest to apply. Gel will add a pretty sheen, and cream blush will leave a very natural-looking glow, but both require careful blending.

COLOR MATCH

Very pale skin looks amazing with a pastel pink shade with cool tones. For skin that is slightly warmer but still pale, look for a pink that is a bit dustier. For skin that tans easily and rarely burns, go with a tawnier pink that has some brown tones in it. Women with tan, warm skin tones should choose an almost plum shade that looks like a rich pink when applied. For deeper skin tones, redder shades that have bluish tones like cranberry leave a beautiful finish.

APPLICATION

Smile and apply powder blush with a brush to the apples of your cheeks, blending out toward the hairline and gently brushing down to blend. Keep blending until the color looks completely natural. Then add a pop of brighter color right on the apples of the cheeks.

For gel or cream blush, apply with your fingers to the apples of the cheeks and up toward the hairline. Apply only a small amount at first and blend thoroughly; you can always add more.

eyeliner

Whether you want to create a dramatic look or just want to make your eyes stand out, liner is the key. Here's everything you need to know.

TYPES

Pencils, powders, gels, pens—liners come in a variety of formulas and each creates a different effect.

PENCIL: Pencil liners are easy to apply. A standard pencil liner creates a very thin, precise line and is good for dry eyelids. If you are looking for something more intense and with a wider line, go with a gel liner pencil. A kajal-formula pencil gives a slightly smudged, sexy look, good for a smoky eye. Longwear pencils will last all day and are the best for warm, humid climates.

GEL: Gel liner provides an intense, crisp line that is smudge-proof, water-resistant, and long-wearing. It comes in a small pot and is applied with a thin brush applicator.

POWDER: Applied with a liner brush, powder liners create a soft line. You can even double up your eye shadow to use as a liner, but powder liner formulas tend to last longer. When applied with a dry brush, the line will be softer. Applying with a slightly damp brush will make a more defined line.

LIQUID: Liquid liner, which comes in a tube with a brush, gives a standout line. It requires some patience and practice to get it right.

APPLICATION

You can try all of these application techniques with all of the different types of liner depending on your desired effect.

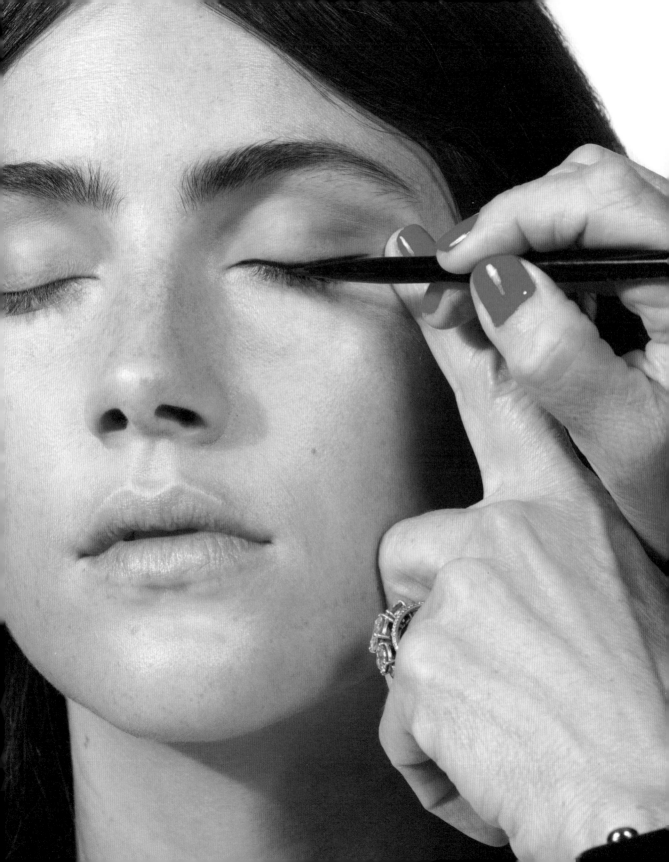

BASIC LINER

To define your eyes and make them pop, all you need is a little liner. Of all the makeup techniques, this is the one people are often intimidated by, but it's easy once you know how.

1. Starting from the outer corner of the eye, line your way across the lashline all the way to the inner corner. Draw the line as close to the lashline as possible.

2. Fill in the line to make it smooth and even and make sure there are no gaps between the liner and lashline.

3. If you want a softer effect, use your finger or a brush to smudge along the lashline.

WINGED LINER

Winged liner adds a little extra drama to the eyes. It can be done with all liner types but is easiest with a pot of gel liner and a thin, tapered brush.

1. Apply liner from the outer corner of the eye all the way across the upper lashline to the inner corner, going thinner with the line as you move toward the inside.

2. To create the wing, extend the line from the outer corner so that it goes up and out, tapering to a soft point. Make sure the wings on both eyes are mirrors of each other.

NOTE: The length of the wing is up to you. You can draw it farther out and straighter or create an upward flick.

LOWER LASH LINER

If you want added definition, try lining the lower lashline, too. I suggest using a darker color on the top lid to create intensity and a more diffused shade underneath.

1. Gel and liquid liner are often too intense for the lower lashline, so use a pencil or powder liner instead. Using a pencil or powder brush, draw a thin line very close to the lashes from the outer corner in.

2. It is important that you connect the upper and lower lines at the outer corner of your eye to help elongate the eye.

NOTE: If you have a lot of undereye darkness, skip this step. A better option is to use waterproof mascara on the lower lashes and skip the liner, as it adds extra darkness.

LAYERING LINER

You can achieve many different effects by layering different liner types. It's fun to play around and see what you like. A thin pencil liner followed by dry powder will create a slightly softer, smudged line. Gel liner on top of a pencil smudged over a powder will create a more intense liner look.

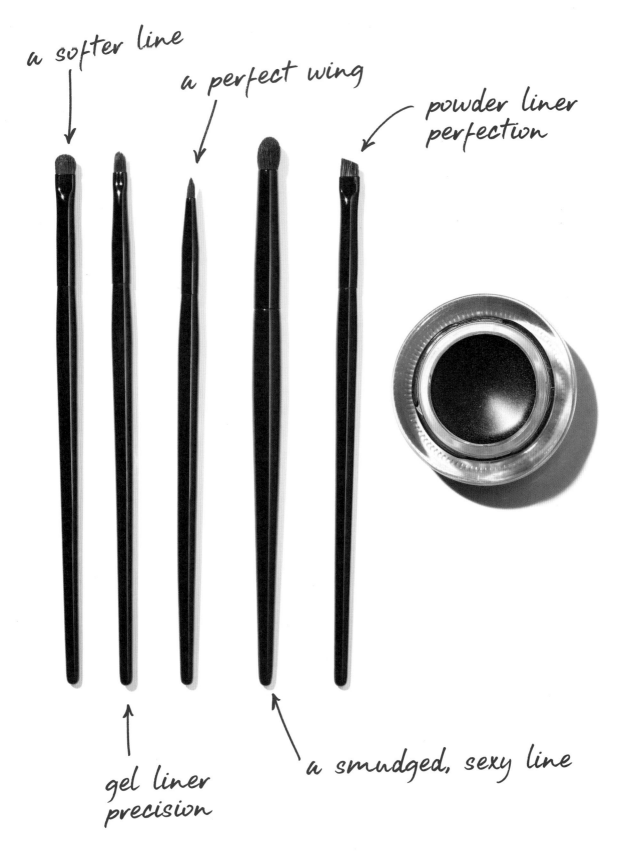

a softer line

a perfect wing

powder liner
perfection

gel liner
precision

a smudged, sexy line

eyeshadow

___

Every woman should have a few go-to shadow combinations, from a pretty, soft shade that opens up the eye to a trio of coordinating deeper shades to create a smoky eye.

TYPES

Powder shadows are the most common and the easiest to apply, layer, and blend. Cream shadows offer more concentrated color and last longer. Powder can be matte, semi-matte, shimmer, glitter, and metallic. Cream shadows can be emollient or even a gloss. Powder shadows can be used to line the eyes and fill in brows. Cream shadows are great for easy application with your finger or a brush and often come in longwear formulas.

COLOR MATCH

There is no one right shadow color. It's really your personal preference. For a basic eye, your base color should be a pale shadow that lightens your whole lid and is almost invisible. I recommend white or bone for fair skin and banana- or peachy-toned shadows for darker skin. Then you can play with medium and darker colors layered on top. If you have redness, stay away from shades with red or purple undertones, as those will highlight the issue.

APPLICATION

There are many ways to apply eyeshadow. It doesn't have to be complicated. I love the look of one gorgeous color paired with black liner and mascara. You can do this with a lighter color to open the eye or a darker color to make a statement.

If you want to create a look with two or three shadows, here's a foolproof way to apply: With an eyeshadow brush, sweep your light base color all over the lid from the lashline up to the brow bone. Apply the medium shadow across the lower lid from the lashline to the crease. You can stop there or add a third, even darker shade in the crease for a smoky eye. The darkest shadow can also be applied as eyeliner using a damp eyeliner brush.

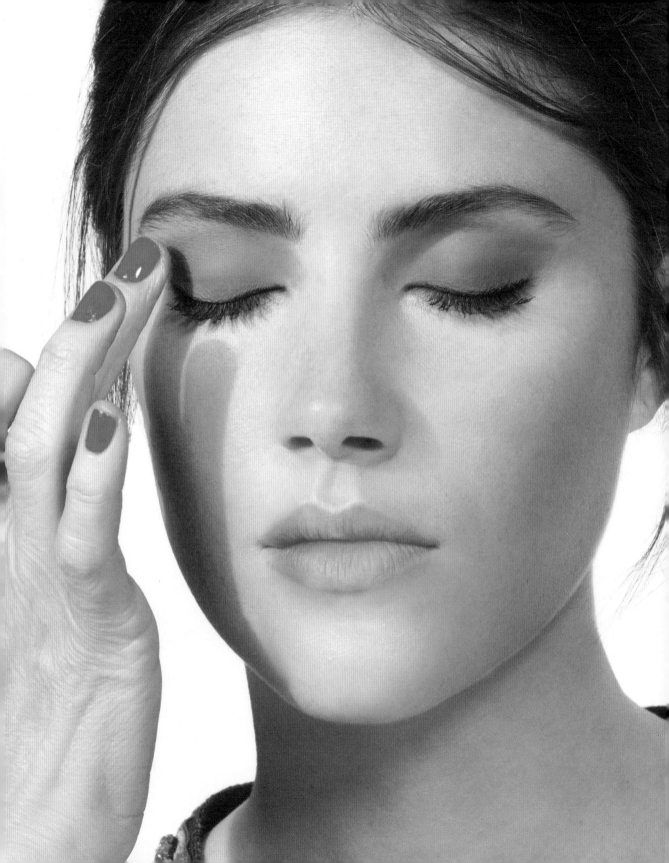

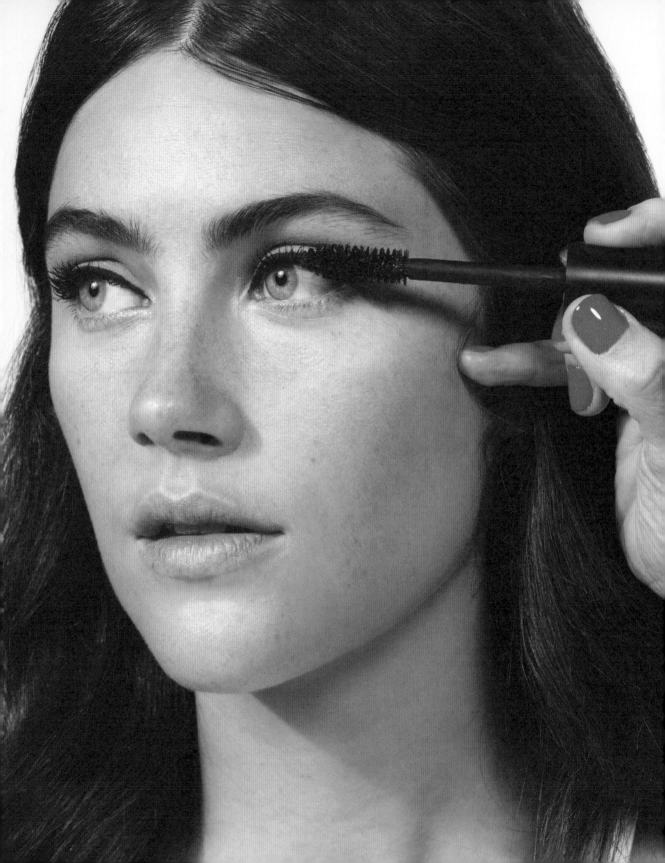

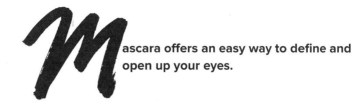

Mascara offers an easy way to define and open up your eyes.

mascara

TYPES

There are many different mascara names and formulas, but they fall into four basic categories. Volumizing and plumping mascaras create the illusion of fuller lashes. Thickening versions bulk up individual lashes. Lengthening elongates lashes. Longwear and waterproof mascaras last the longest, holding product from day to night.

COLOR MATCH

The one shade of mascara that looks good on everyone is black. If you are blonde or have light red hair, dark brown is an option, but only if you want a more subtle, natural look. Otherwise, choose the blackest mascara you can find and wear it day and night.

APPLICATION

Always begin by putting mascara on the top lashes, coating the entire lash. Apply one or two coats for a natural look, three for more definition. Bottom lashes need only one coat.

Layering different mascara formulas works to get the benefits of each. Apply a couple coats of one formula, let it dry for a minute, and then follow with a few coats of the second formula. (The order in which you apply the different formulas doesn't matter—you'll still get the effects from both.)

your best lip

Every woman should have a natural shade of lipstick that she can swipe on without looking in the mirror. Using different colors and formulas is a fun, quick way to change up your look.

TYPES

Formula is everything when it comes to lipstick. Creamy formulas offer hydrating semi-matte coverage in a creamy finish. Matte lipsticks offer dense, matte, long-lasting finish. Sheer versions offer a transparent wash of your favorite shade. Gloss offers moisturizing benefits with a shiny finish. Use a gloss on its own for a touch of color or layered on top of a lipstick for some added sheen. Chubby lip pencils add definition and long-lasting color. Lip liners help define lips with a thin line of lasting color around or underneath your lipstick.

COLOR MATCH

The right lip color for you is based on three things: your style, your natural lip color, and your skin tone.

To find your best nude—your go-to color for an everyday, natural lip—shop when you are barefaced. Bite your lips and then try to find a lipstick that matches that color. The right shade will give your complexion a lift and make your eyes appear brighter—even when it's all you have on. In general, the most flattering natural hue will either match or be slightly darker than your lips. Avoid shades lighter than your lips, especially those with gray or beige undertones, as they will make you look washed out.

If you want to make a statement, go with strong colors like classic red, deep burgundy, or bright orange. Don't be afraid to mix your own shade, using two or more of your favorite colors. I never choose a lipstick color to match clothes; instead I like to keep a balance and avoid a color war. If you are wearing strong colors, your lips can be more neutral and vice versa. Bright pink lip? Go with navy, gray, or white for your top.

APPLICATION

Whether you use a lip brush or apply straight out of the tube, make sure lip color is within the natural lines of your lips. A brush allows a more precise application that works really well with stronger colors. There isn't one way to apply lipstick. You can apply the color all over both lips or just on the bottom lip and then rub the two together. You can also blot a small amount and pair it with gloss to make it more of a stain. Lip liner can be applied all over lips, underneath lipstick, for longer-lasting color. Or it can be applied after lipstick (but make sure the liner matches your lip color).

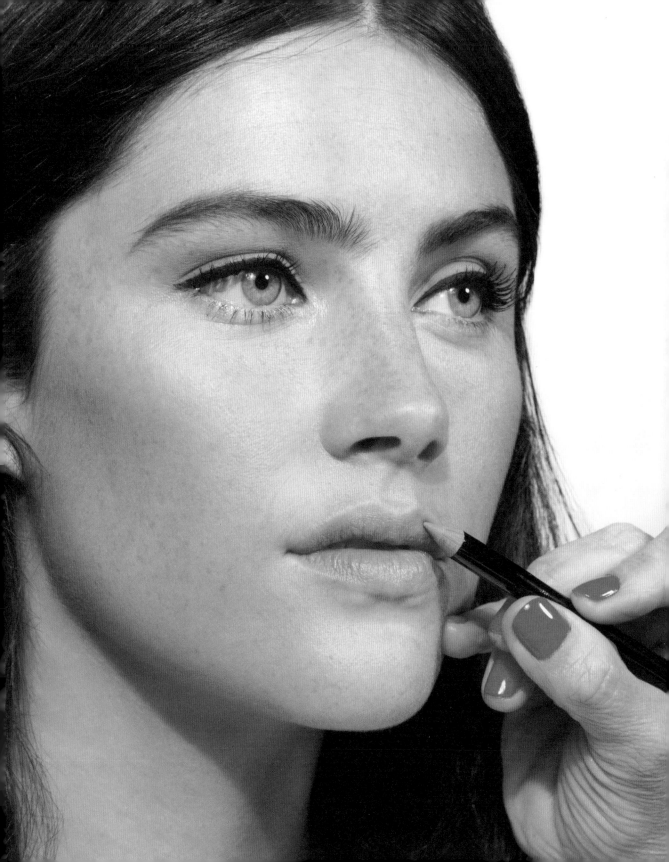

BROWS 101

Brows are often ignored, but a beautifully defined pair has the power to transform your look. The right shape and definition can balance out your features and frame your eyes. Follow these steps.

BRUSH UP your brows with a brow brush.

TRIM brows with small brow scissors if you have stray hairs growing outside your brow shape.

TWEEZE any stray brow hairs. Try to follow the natural shape of your brows. Don't overtweeze, as super-thin brows aren't flattering on anyone. It is helpful to get a professional to shape your brows and then maintain the shape on your own.

DEFINE your brows by filling in any bare areas with a brush and eye shadow or brow powder, or a pencil. Choose a shade in the same tone as your brow color. If you have black hair, go with a slightly softer shade, like a dark ash brown or a deep brown-black. If you are blonde, keep the shadow in the same tone as your brow hair. Fill in starting at the inner corner of your brows and brush straight up. For the rest of the brow, brush up and over along the shape of your brow, filling in any gaps with powder. If you still have bare spots, try filling them in with an eyeliner pencil.

TAME unruly brows using clear brow shaper. The product comes with a wand that you brush into your brows to apply a clear gel.

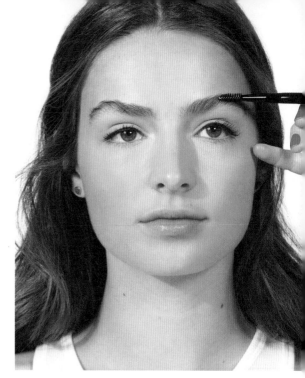

1. brush up

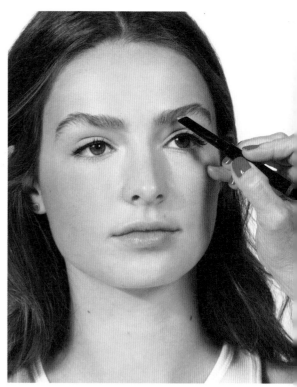

4. fill in with pencil

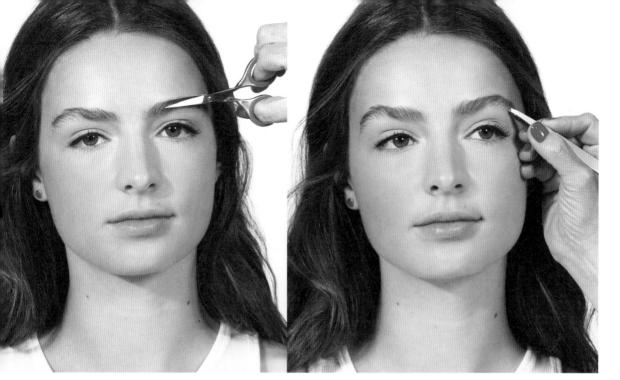

2. trim

3. tweeze

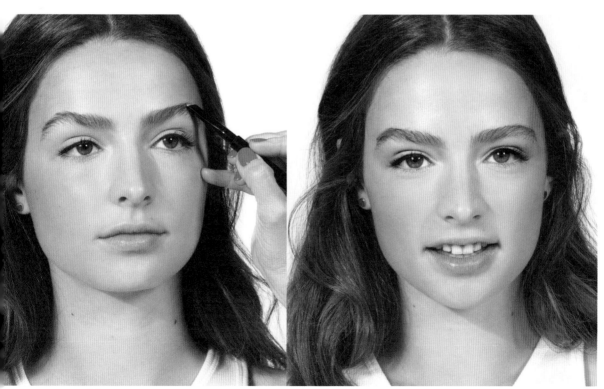

5. fill up to arch

6. voilà

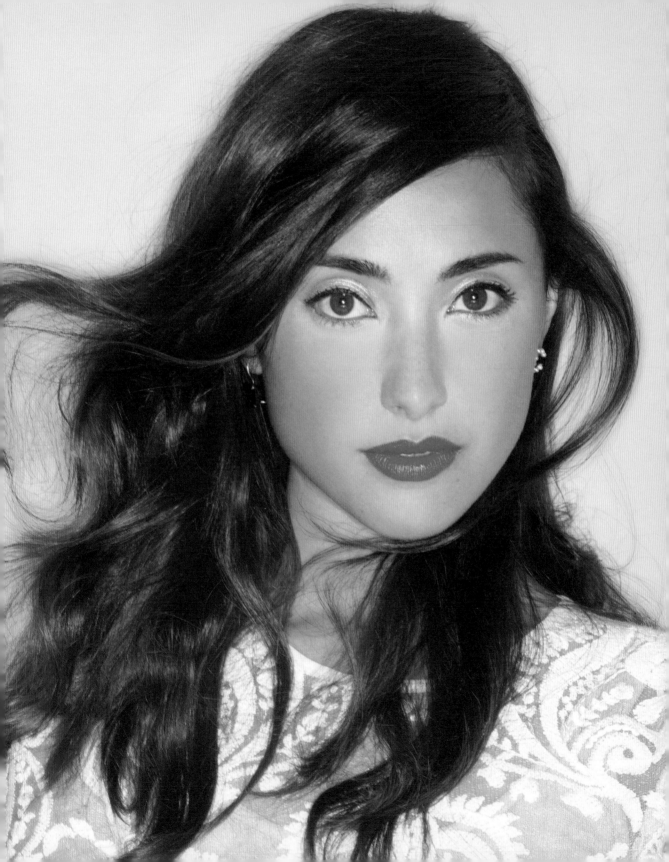

Mix Up Your Look

Once you've mastered the basics, it's time to break the rules. You don't always have to do your makeup the same way—there are too many amazing techniques, formulas, and colors to stick to only one combination. Skin looks great? Skip foundation. Want an easy new look for your lips? Throw a shimmery blush stick on your cheeks and pat some on your lips, too. Go with highlighting powder on your cheekbones and smudge some on your eyelids and then top with mascara. Be open and try new things. Here are some simple and modern ways to be inspired.

cool makeup looks

Switch it up. Don't stick with the same look forever because it's safe or easy. Every few months you should play with new palettes or techniques. Just trying one new move, one cool color, or a different finish can make a big impact.

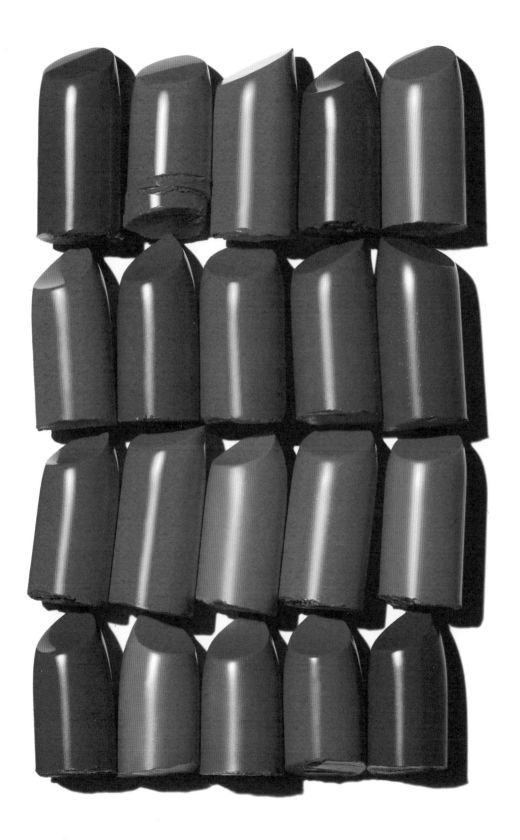

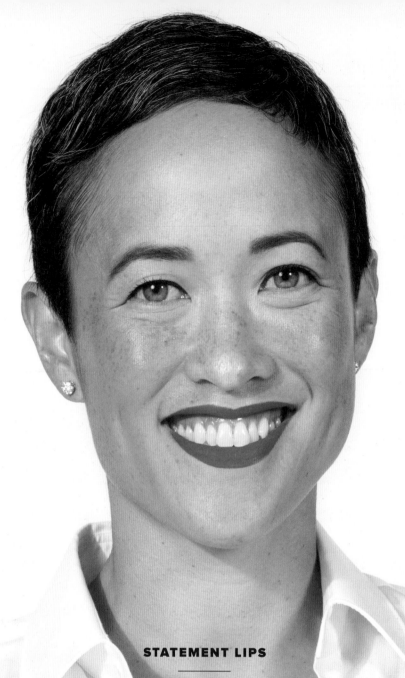

STATEMENT LIPS

I love the combo of a crisp white shirt, minimal makeup, and bold red lips. Tinted moisturizer paired with concealer leaves a dewy, even finish on skin. Rosy cream blush blended on apples of cheeks adds a little color. Espresso gel liner applied very close to the top lashline topped with black mascara subtly defines eyes, while red lips steal the spotlight.

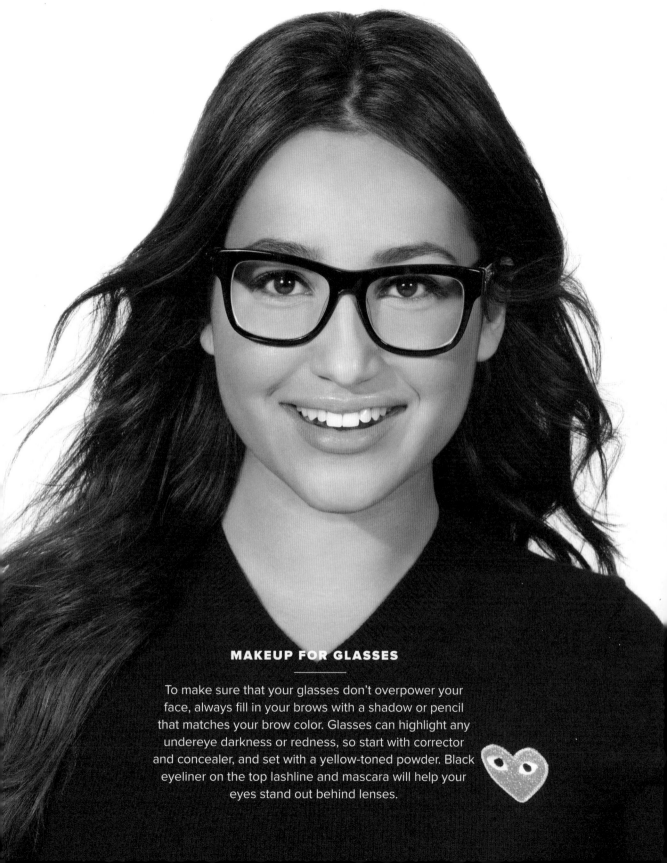

MAKEUP FOR GLASSES

To make sure that your glasses don't overpower your face, always fill in your brows with a shadow or pencil that matches your brow color. Glasses can highlight any undereye darkness or redness, so start with corrector and concealer, and set with a yellow-toned powder. Black eyeliner on the top lashline and mascara will help your eyes stand out behind lenses.

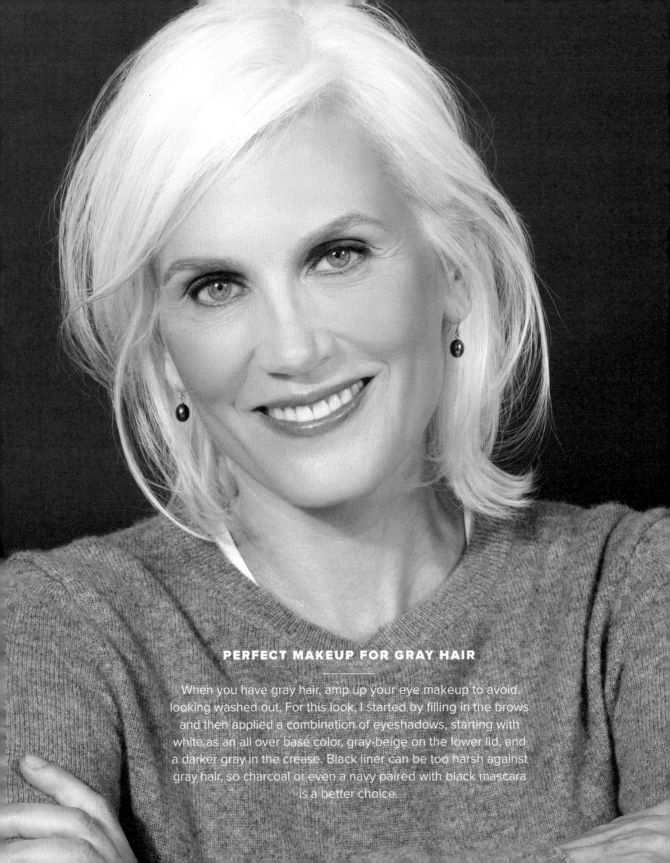

PERFECT MAKEUP FOR GRAY HAIR

When you have gray hair, amp up your eye makeup to avoid
looking washed out. For this look, I started by filling in the brows
and then applied a combination of eyeshadows, starting with
white as an all over base color, gray-beige on the lower lid, and
a darker gray in the crease. Black liner can be too harsh against
gray hair, so charcoal or even a navy paired with black mascara
is a better choice.

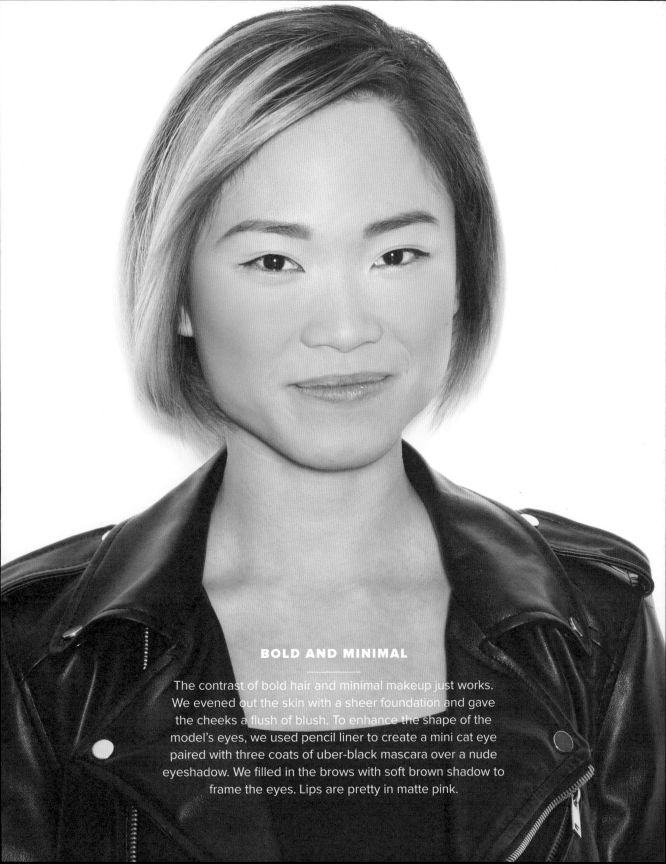

BOLD AND MINIMAL

The contrast of bold hair and minimal makeup just works. We evened out the skin with a sheer foundation and gave the cheeks a flush of blush. To enhance the shape of the model's eyes, we used pencil liner to create a mini cat eye paired with three coats of uber-black mascara over a nude eyeshadow. We filled in the brows with soft brown shadow to frame the eyes. Lips are pretty in matte pink.

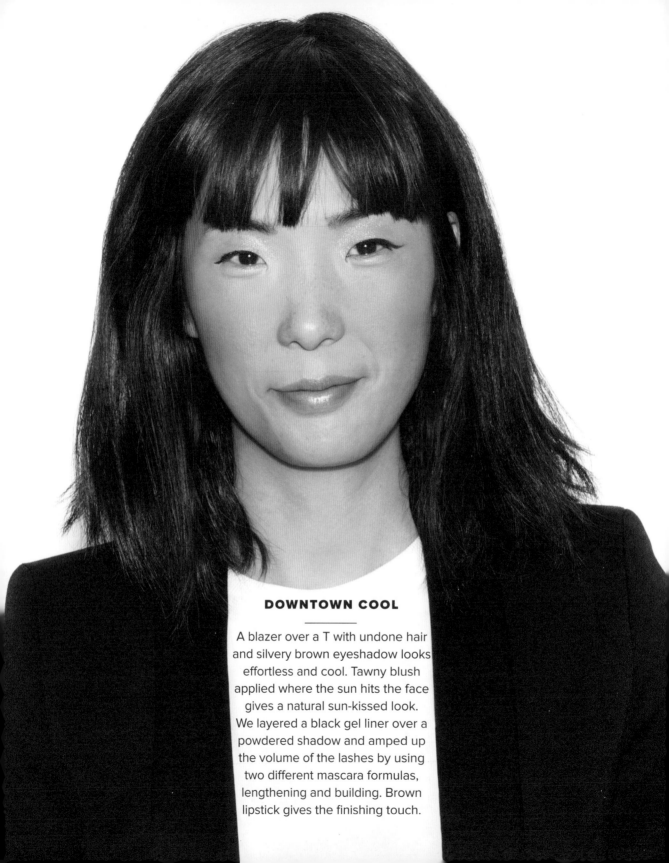

DOWNTOWN COOL

A blazer over a T with undone hair and silvery brown eyeshadow looks effortless and cool. Tawny blush applied where the sun hits the face gives a natural sun-kissed look. We layered a black gel liner over a powdered shadow and amped up the volume of the lashes by using two different mascara formulas, lengthening and building. Brown lipstick gives the finishing touch.

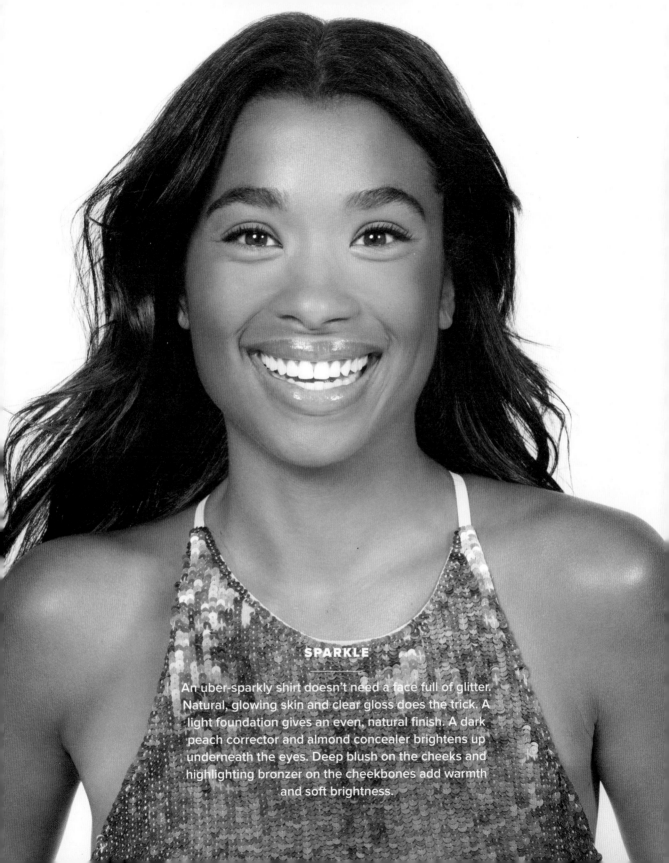

SPARKLE

An uber-sparkly shirt doesn't need a face full of glitter. Natural, glowing skin and clear gloss does the trick. A light foundation gives an even, natural finish. A dark peach corrector and almond concealer brightens up underneath the eyes. Deep blush on the cheeks and highlighting bronzer on the cheekbones add warmth and soft brightness.

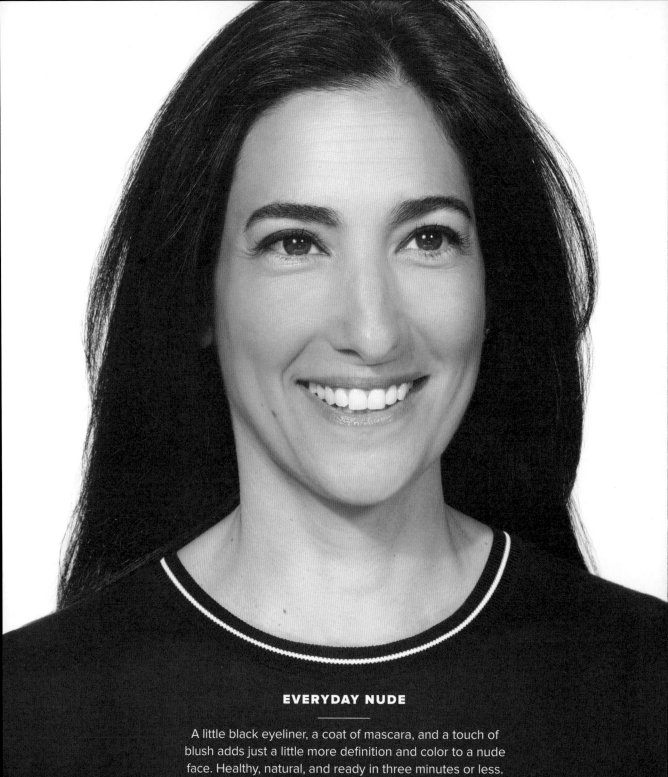

EVERYDAY NUDE

A little black eyeliner, a coat of mascara, and a touch of
blush adds just a little more definition and color to a nude
face. Healthy, natural, and ready in three minutes or less.

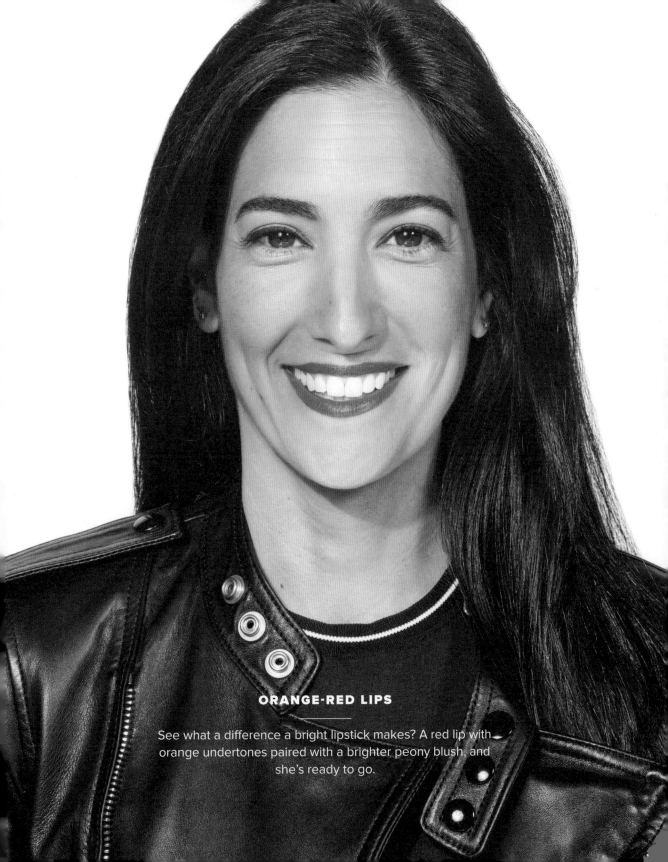

ORANGE-RED LIPS

See what a difference a bright lipstick makes? A red lip with orange undertones paired with a brighter peony blush, and she's ready to go.

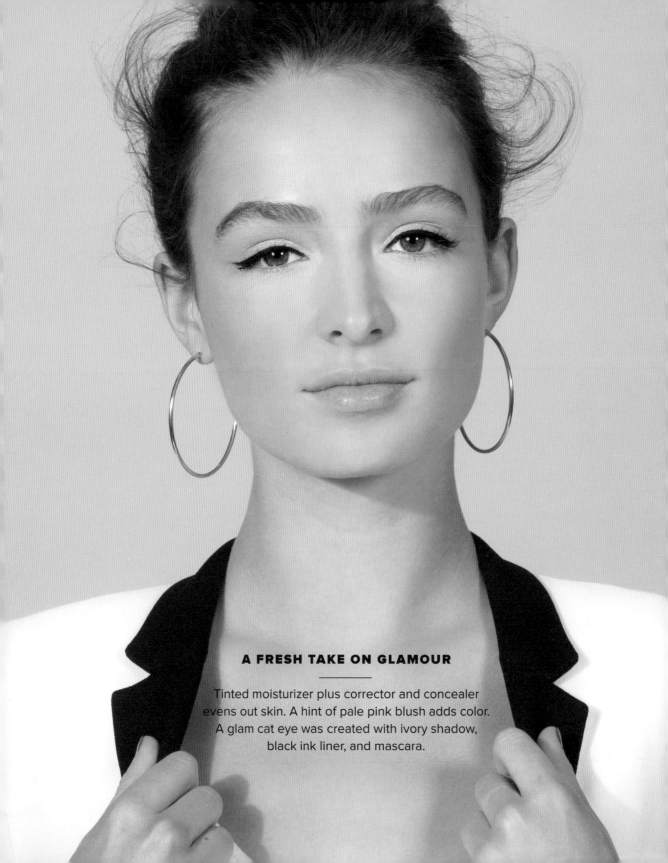

A FRESH TAKE ON GLAMOUR

Tinted moisturizer plus corrector and concealer
evens out skin. A hint of pale pink blush adds color.
A glam cat eye was created with ivory shadow,
black ink liner, and mascara.

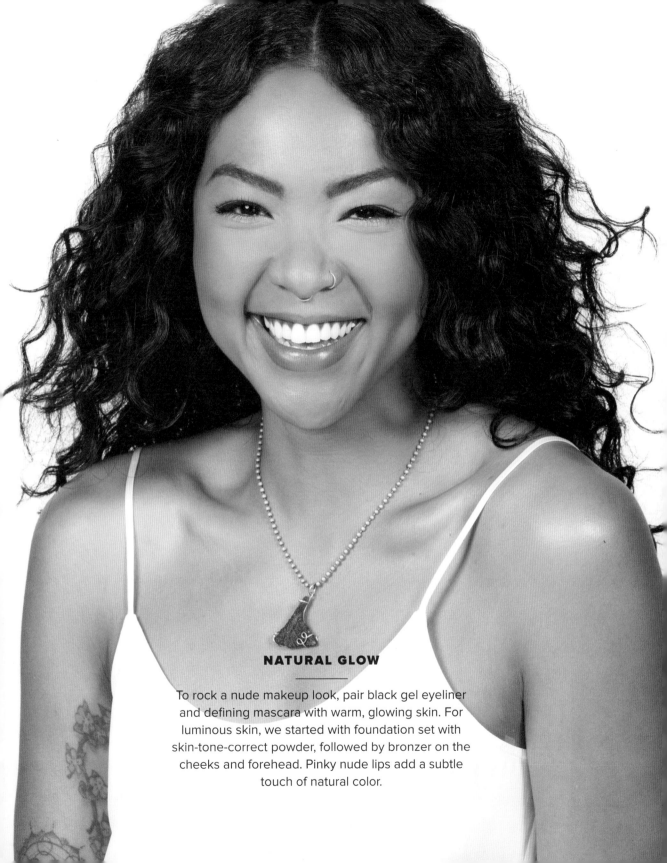

NATURAL GLOW

To rock a nude makeup look, pair black gel eyeliner
and defining mascara with warm, glowing skin. For
luminous skin, we started with foundation set with
skin-tone-correct powder, followed by bronzer on the
cheeks and forehead. Pinky nude lips add a subtle
touch of natural color.

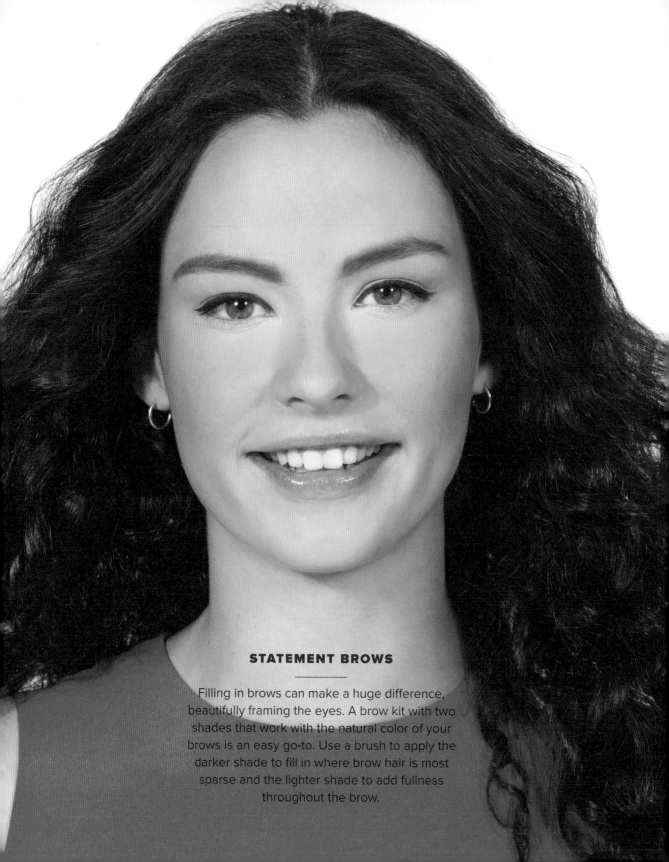

STATEMENT BROWS

Filling in brows can make a huge difference, beautifully framing the eyes. A brow kit with two shades that work with the natural color of your brows is an easy go-to. Use a brush to apply the darker shade to fill in where brow hair is most sparse and the lighter shade to add fullness throughout the brow.

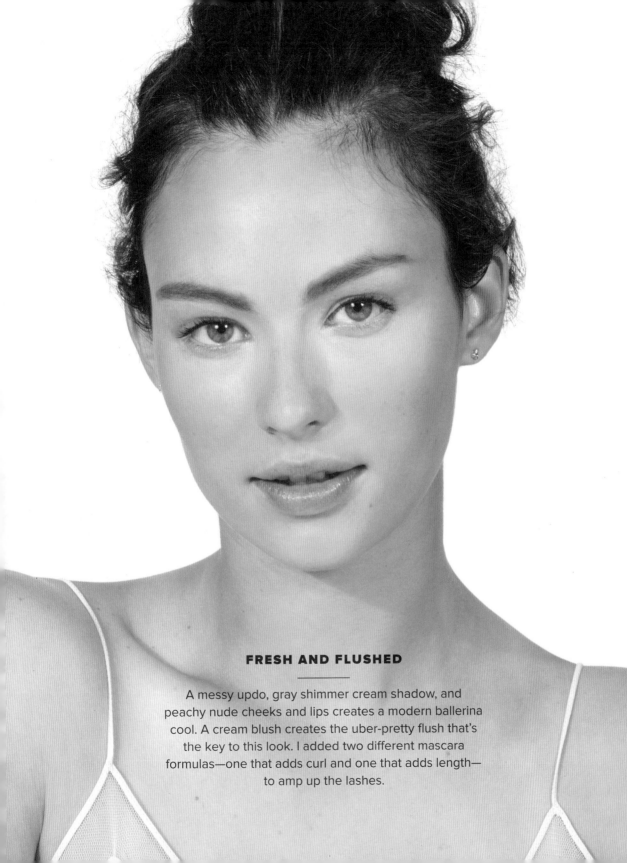

FRESH AND FLUSHED

A messy updo, gray shimmer cream shadow, and
peachy nude cheeks and lips creates a modern ballerina
cool. A cream blush creates the uber-pretty flush that's
the key to this look. I added two different mascara
formulas—one that adds curl and one that adds length—
to amp up the lashes.

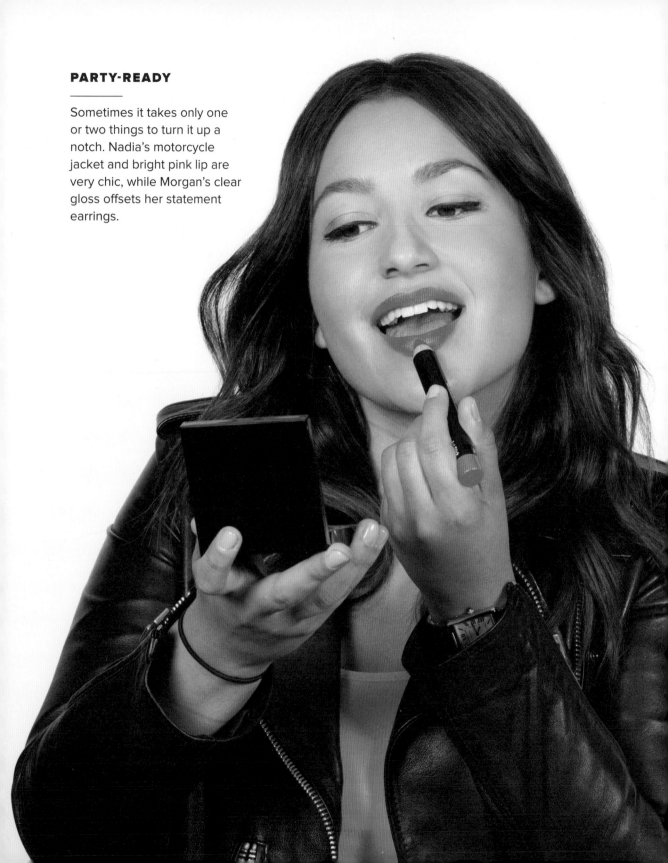

PARTY-READY

Sometimes it takes only one or two things to turn it up a notch. Nadia's motorcycle jacket and bright pink lip are very chic, while Morgan's clear gloss offsets her statement earrings.

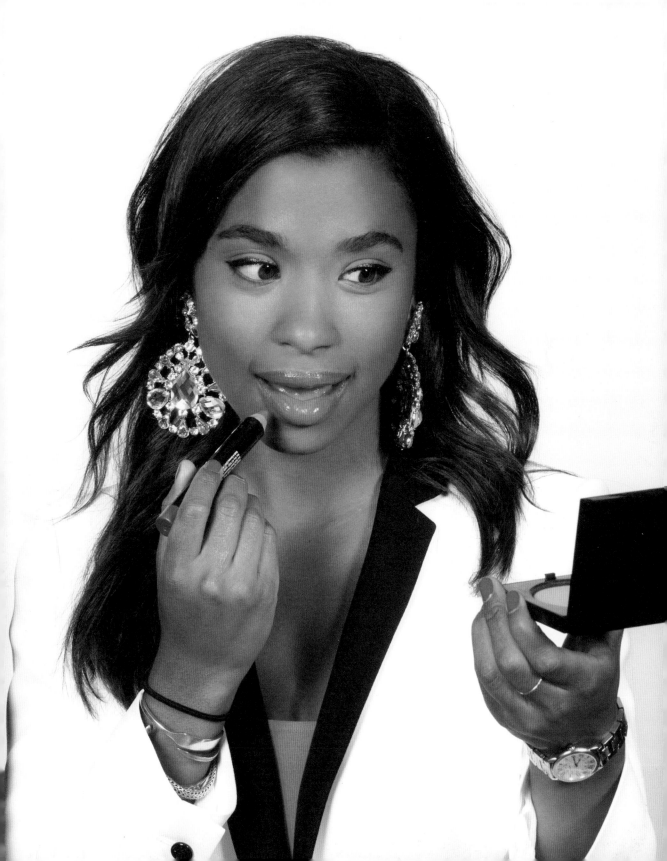

makeovers

Women look beautiful with and without makeup. New products, different techniques, and different palettes can change up your look in subtle or high-impact ways. Get inspired by these looks.

VERONICA

For a natural, even finish, you can correct any unevenness with stick foundation. Just spot correct where needed; on Veronica I did touches around the mouth and on her forehead. I also played up her naturally strong brows by filling them in with a matching pencil and layering with shadow. Deep berry blush and lips pull it all together.

KATHERINE

Just a few subtle changes add up to a totally different look. Start by taking strands from straight to slightly wavy with a hot iron. To create flawless skin with a matte finish, use corrector and concealer set with yellow powder underneath eyes and foundation set with skin-tone-correct powder for face. Brush up brows up with a brush, choose a shadow that matches your brow color, fill in with a shadow brush, and set with a brow gel. Cream eye shadow applied all over the lids and black mascara finishes the eyes. For a precise red lip, apply color with a lip brush.

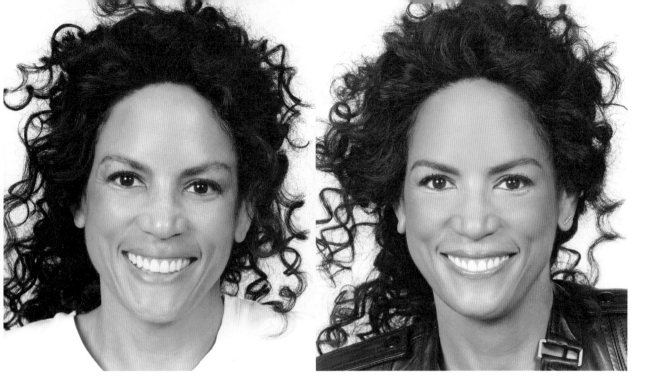

Veronica

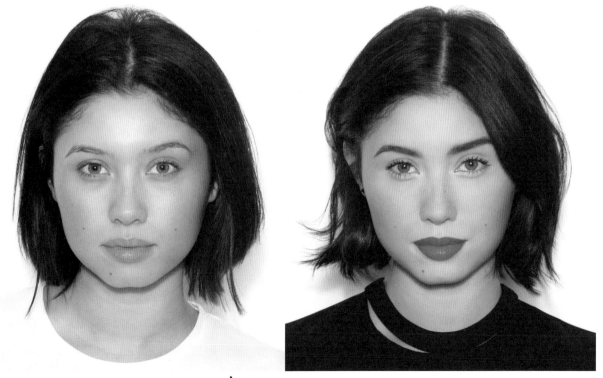

Katherine

DIANE

The cool shape and pale pink hue make these glasses unexpected, so makeup can take a backseat. But defining the eyes underneath statement frames is essential. Here we did a very thin, yet intense, gel liner applied with a brush very close to the upper lashline. This enhances her eye shape and makes sure her eyes don't get lost behind her glasses.

ANIA

Take away any redness in skin with a yellow-toned tinted moisturizer. Then, touch up with a foundation stick to ensure that skin is even but still fresh. Here I added tone-correcting loose powder to set the makeup so it lasts and keeps redness away. I defined eyes with a navy line over grayish taupe eyeshadow and filled in her brows at the same time. I brought color to the face with rosy pink lips and matching blush. A modern blowout frames her face perfectly.

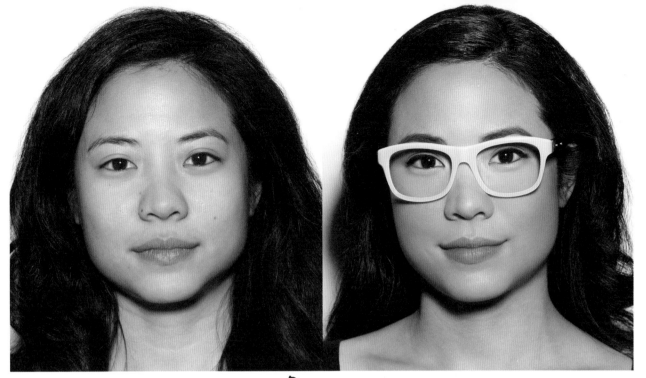

Diane

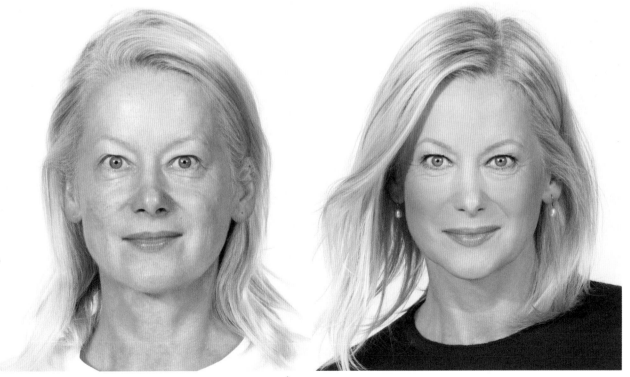

Ania

Jessica

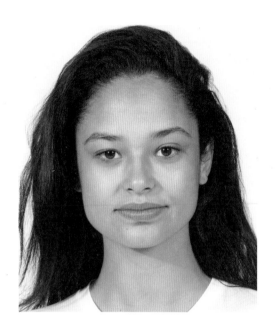

INTENSE LINER

For a stronger eye look, line eyes with pencil all the way around. Make sure the line gets wider and thicker as it goes to the outer corner. Creamy skin and pretty pink blush balance it all out.

BOLD LIP

I love a bold lip with tinted moisturizer, pink blush, mascara, and a touch of shimmer shadow. For statement red lips, go with bright pink or blue-red on very pale skin. For warmer skin tones, try an orange-red. Deep skin tones look great in a browner red. Opt for a creamy semi-matte or a true matte finish for long-lasting wear, but make sure the formula isn't too dry or it will noticeably dry out lips. Apply with a brush and blot with a tissue for a precise, even finish.

GLASSES

You want your eyes to stand out underneath your frames. A smoky eye in brown or bronzy shades looks pretty underneath tortoise rims.

CAT EYE

If you want to amp up your eyes, apply a slightly thicker line over your daytime liner. A gel liner applied with a brush works best. Extend out from the outer corner up and out to a fine point. A cat eye looks current paired with nude lips and a barely there color on cheeks.

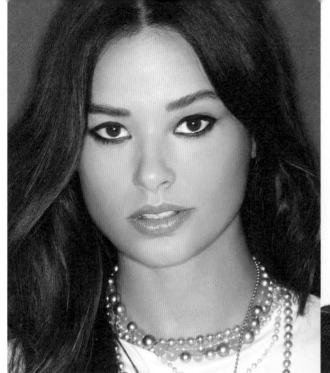

intense liner

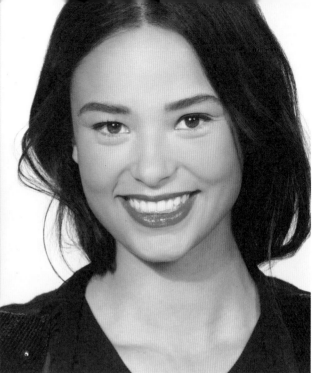

bold lip

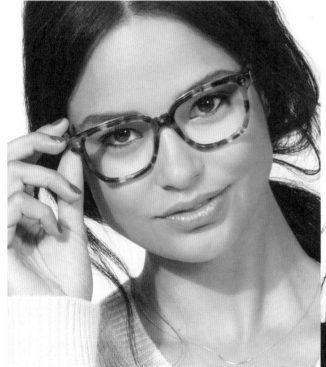

glasses

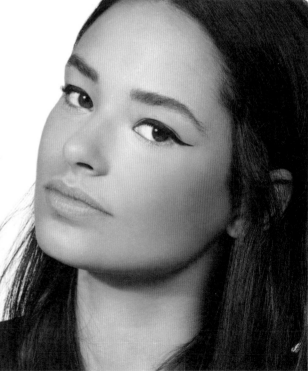

cat eye

Anna

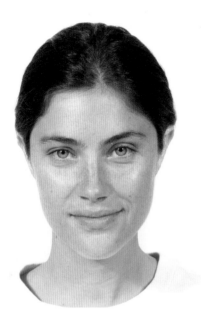

forehead gives a glow to the face. This highlighting technique is called strobing. It looks great with a simple eye (just liner and mascara) and a pretty nude lip, like Anna's pinky rose shade.

SIMPLE SMOKY EYE

Want an easier way to do a smoky eye? Go with cream shadows. They are easier to blend and apply. To get this look, use an ivory cream shadow stick all over the lids, then add a deep gray-purple into the entire crease, and slate in the outer corner. Using a smudging brush, apply a thin line of greige shadow to line the lower lashline. Charcoal gel liner on the top lashline and black volumizing mascara finish the look. A nude lip and dusty pink blush keep the focus on the eyes. For an effortless take on the updo, try a middle part, and keep it slightly undone and imperfect.

PRETTY IN PINK

To dress up a graphic sweatshirt, go with the unexpected pairing of layered pearls offset with a chic, messy side pony. A pinky peach cheek and lip on top of glowing skin looks just right.

GLOW

Your makeup should reflect your style. This look is the perfect combo of sporty and cool. Cream blush combined with highlighting powder placed high on the cheekbones and lightly dusted across the

CLASSIC

A crisp button-down white shirt always works, and makeup doesn't have to be complicated, either. Here, soft gray shadow and black mascara complement a filled-in brow. A nude pink blush and lip are simple and elegant. Loosen up the look with natural, wavy hair.

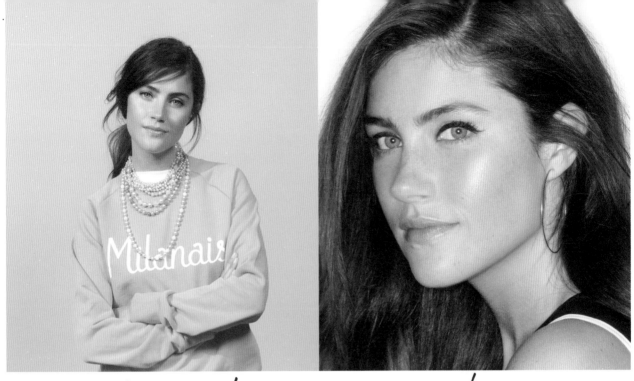

pretty in pink

glow

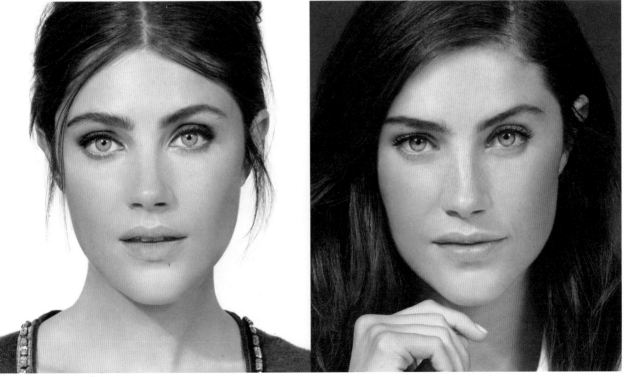

simple smoky eye

classic

Mollye

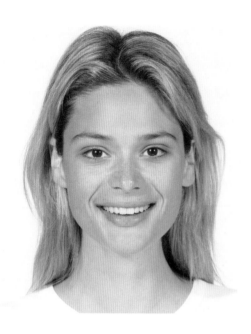

CLASSIC

When you want a more polished look, keep it classic with a combo of white, gray, and slate eye shadows paired with a creamy pink lip. To create well-defined brows, brush them up with a brow brush, choose a shadow that matches your brow color, fill in with a shadow brush, then finish with a brow gel. A middle part with front strands clipped together in back is a simple way to pull together long wavy hair.

MOD

For a mod '60s look, even out the skin with a foundation stick and try a beige lipstick. This pale lip color works because it is not too white and has a hint of pink. Thanks to well-defined eyes and bright pink cheeks, she looks cool, not washed out. Bonus points for face-framing bangs.

HIGH GLOSS

Eyegloss is a product developed straight from the runway, but it still looks cool in real life. You will need even skin for this look, so spot treat redness with a corrector, followed by a concealer and foundation stick. Sweep nude/rose eyeshadow on the lids, followed by soft smudged chocolate liner on the top lashline. Apply eyegloss to lids using your fingers, and add a clear lip gloss on lips to balance out the look.

SLEEK

The red lip stain and sleek take on the classic pony looks sophisticated and modern. For hair, start with pin-straight hair (you may need to use a hair-straightening balm and a flat iron first), then create a deep side part and pull hair into a smooth and low ponytail.

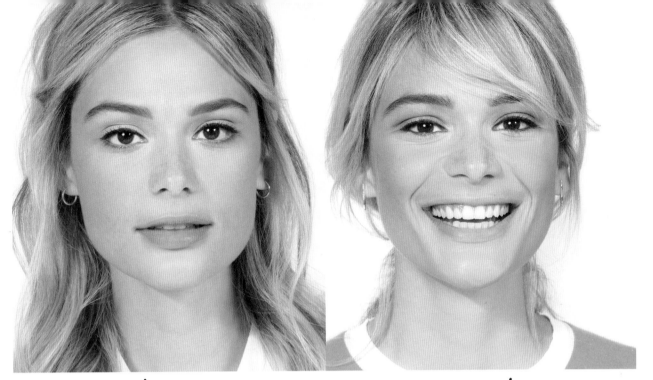

classic

mod

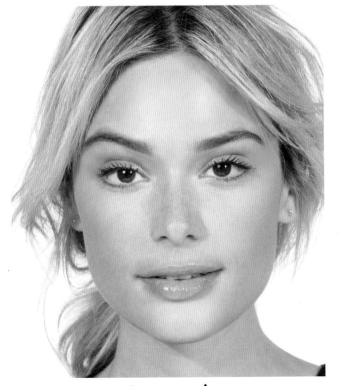

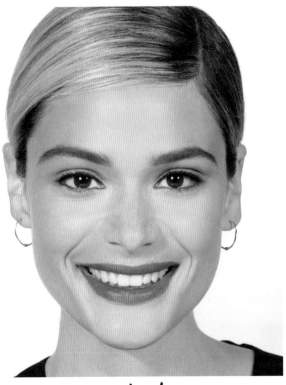

high gloss

sleek

Sarmishta

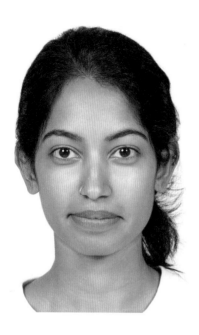

MATTE

Sleek, pin-straight hair in a middle part gives a retro *Love Story*–inspired hair look. Subtle makeup keeps the focus on her striking hair.

READY IN FIVE

Tinted moisturizer hydrates, evens out, and protects skin with SPF. Eye cream followed by corrector, concealer, and mascara brightens and opens up the eye. A berry blush adds a pretty, natural flush.

BOLD LIP

Bold lips were made for a night out. For more intensity, try darker reds like this deep burgundy shade. For color that will stay on all night, a lip pencil has longer staying power than a lipstick.

SUBTLE SHINE

Build on the five-minute look by adding liner to top lashes, volumizing mascara, a creamy nude lip color, and highlighter placed high on cheekbones.

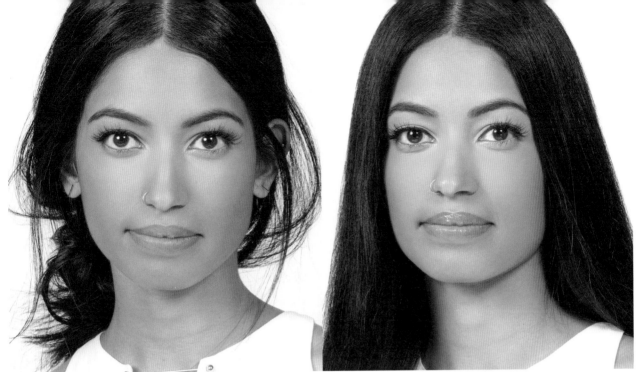

subtle shine

matte

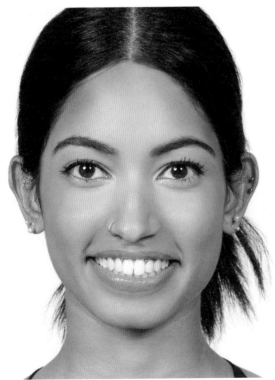

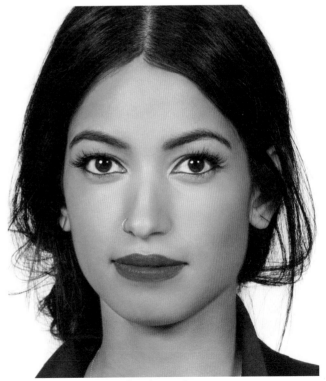

ready in five

bold lip

a big thank-you to:

My biggest thank-you is to my husband and my sons, who support me and always keep me on my toes.

Team Bobbi
Steven Plofker
Sara Bliss
Tara Tersigni
Roza Israel
John Eaton
Kim Soane
Cassandra Garcia
Yuby Leoce
Hannah Martin
Mallory McLoughlin
Alexis Rodriguez
Alex Perron
Lila Claghorn
Hervé Claude Bernard
Amerinda Callahan
Derek Brahney
Studio 042
Lauren Larco
Jill Velez
Lily Becker
Julie Borowsky
Sloane Schmitt

Photographers
Ben Ritter
Jon Paterson
Sarah Elliott

Photo Assistants
Natalia Mantini
Alex Jiang

Chronicle Books
Christine Carswell
Pamela Geismar
Laura Lee Mattingly
Sara Waitt
Yolanda Cazares
Alexandra Brown

The Experts
Dr. Charles Passler
Summer Ashley Singletary
Sarah Kate Benjamin
Daryl Gioffre
Mila Moursi
Dr. Frank Lipman
Tracie Martyn
Dr. Shirley Madhere
Dr. Sejal Shah
Charlie Knoles
Kelly Stackhouse
Lily Kunin
Dr. Robin Berzin
Harley Pasternak
David Kirsch
Ashley Wilking
Shom Chowdhury
Jen Kluczkowski
Dr. Jeff Lally, D.C.
Amy Galper
Dr. Macrene Alexiades
Dr. Amy Shah
Dr. Ken Davis
Lauren Slayton
Dr. Rosemarie Ingleton
Tricia Williams
Cody Plofker

Models
Hannah Bronfman
Gabby Reece

Laila Ali
Maye Musk
Cassandra Grey
Elle Macpherson
Olivia Munn
Veronica Webb
Sarmishta Mahendra
Anna Speckhart
Mollye Rogel
Jessica Pott
Alyssa Reeder
Kristen Weavers
Sam Gold
Kelly Stackhouse
Ania Morehand
Kim Santacruz
Marie Claire Katigbak
Nadia Morehand
Morgan Booker
Mai Kato
Giang Vo
Katherine Ross
Glynnis Harvey
Diane Duong

Casting
Christian Meshesha
Steven Williams

The Studios
18 Label Studios
Liz Sardinsky

Our Caterers
Falafel Hut
Jane Yagoda

The Transportation
Starlane Car & Limousine
    Service

INDEX

STOP OBSESSING ABOUT YOUR FLAWS

FOCUS ON WHAT YOU DO LIKE

WEAR BLUSH

MOVE YOUR BODY EVERY DAY

BE NICE

HELP SOMEONE

HIGHLIGHT THE POSITIVE

TRY A NEW FOOD

PUT CUCUMBER IN YOUR WATER

PUT A LITTLE COCONUT OIL IN YOUR HAIR

MASTER THE SMOKY EYE